国家心血管病中心
中国医学科学院阜外医院
心血管外科年度报告2022

主 编 胡盛寿

National Center For Cardiovascular Diseases

Fuwai Hospital, Chinese Academy of Medical Sciences, Peking Union Medical College

CARDIOVASCULAR SURGERY

OUTCOMES 2022

中国协和医科大学出版社

北 京

图书在版编目（CIP）数据

国家心血管病中心中国医学科学院阜外医院心血管外科年度报告. 2022 / 胡盛寿主编. — 北京：中国协和医科大学出版社，2023.8

ISBN 978－7－5679－2234－1

Ⅰ.①国…　Ⅱ.①胡…　Ⅲ.①心脏外科学－研究报告－北京－2022 ②血管外科学－研究报告－北京－2022　Ⅳ.①R654

中国国家版本馆CIP数据核字（2023）第134460号

国家心血管病中心中国医学科学院阜外医院心血管外科年度报告2022

主　　编：胡盛寿
责任编辑：李元君　胡安霞
封面设计：邱晓俐
责任校对：张　麓
责任印制：张　岱

出版发行：**中国协和医科大学出版社**
　　　　　（北京市东城区东单三条9号　邮编100730　电话010-65260431）
网　　址：www.pumcp.com
经　　销：新华书店总店北京发行所
印　　刷：小森印刷（北京）有限公司

开　　本：889mm×1194mm　　1/16
印　　张：4.75
字　　数：110千字
版　　次：2023年8月第1版
印　　次：2023年8月第1次印刷
定　　价：120.00元

ISBN 978－7－5679－2234－1

编者名单

主　编　胡盛寿

副主编　郑　哲　赵　韡　袁　昕

编　者　袁　靖　陈　凯　储　庆　高仕君

　　　　　饶辰飞　罗明尧　马　凯　徐心仪

　　　　　王玉鑫　陈蔚南　陈　轩

院长寄语
President's address

尊敬的广大同仁及患者朋友们，

大家好！

岁月不居，时节如流，中国医学科学院阜外医院（简称"阜外医院"）2022年外科年报与各位如期相会。在过去的一年里，阜外医院外科同仁们全面贯彻党的二十大精神，聚焦于"推进健康中国建设"任务，全心全意为患者提供优质的医疗服务。在国内新冠疫情肆虐、国际竞争形势加剧的大背景下，外科同仁们坚持问题目标导向，立足中心－医院工作实际，抓住机遇，直面挑战，进一步提高医疗质量，加强创新技术引领，在心血管外科行业内交出了满意的答卷。

在兼顾医疗规模与医疗质量的同时，阜外医院外科以信息化为抓手，持续推进以大数据为支撑的医院信息化、智能化、网络化、自动化建设。依托医院"智慧化"信息系统和全程医疗服务平台，外科同仁们在保证疾病救治工作对标国际先进水平的同时，切实推进健康管理、疾病预防和术后康复工作的发展，将医疗工作的重点从治疗疾病投射到"健康管理－预防－治疗－康复"的全生命周期医疗服务上来。

时值党的二十大的开局之年，我们将以"三个转变、三个提高"为核心，秉持"品质与创新"理念，着力提升内涵建设水平，努力将公立医院推向更高质量、高水平发展，做出高度！

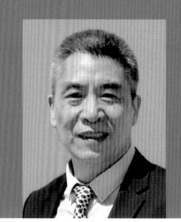

Dear colleagues and patients，

I'm glad that the Fuwai Surgery Outcomes meets our colleagues and patients as promised. In 2022, surgical colleagues in Fuwai Hospital have fully implemented the spirit of the 20th CPC National Congress, focused on the task of "promoting the construction of a healthy China", and wholeheartedly provided the best quality medical services for patients. Under the background of the increasing international competition, surgical colleagues in various fields seize the opportunities, face the challenges, improve medical quality dutifully, strengthen innovation and lead technological development, and continue to take the lead in the cardiovascular surgery industry.

While taking into account the scale and quality of medical care, surgical colleagues promoted the construction of hospital informatization, intelligence, networking and automation supported by big data. Relying on the hospital's "intelligent information system" and the "whole-process medical service department", surgical colleagues, while ensuring the international-advanced level of disease treatment, earnestly promoted the development of health management, disease prevention and postoperative rehabilitation, and projected the focus of medical work from the treatment of diseases to the full life cycle medical service of "health management-prevention-treatment-rehabilitation".

In the year of the 20th CPC National Congress, we will take "three changes and three improvements" as the core and uphold the concept of "quality and innovation". We promise to promote national medical progress and medical service capacity.

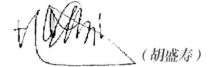 （胡盛寿）

中国工程院院士
国家心血管病中心主任
中国医学科学院阜外医院院长

Shengshou Hu

Academician of Chinese Academy of Engineering
Director of National Center for Cardiovascular Diseases
President of Fuwai Hospital, CAMS&PUMC

目 录
Table of Contents

OUTCOMES 2022

医疗品质
QUALITY OF CARE

一、概况
Overview

　　根据《基本医疗卫生与健康促进法》和国务院出台"十四五"专项规划的要求，阜外医院积极贯彻"双中心"战略部署，目前已形成一个国家中心、三个区域分中心的模式。中国医学科学院阜外医院作为国家医学中心，阜外华中心血管病医院、深圳阜外心血管病医院、云南阜外心血管病医院等作为区域医疗中心，实现了"双中心"战略布局。

　　阜外医院各中心深入开展核心技术攻关，着力解决影响人民健康的长期性、全局性医学问题。对于完善我国医疗服务体系、引领医学科学发展和整体医疗服务能力提升，具有十分重大的战略意义。

　　2022年，四地阜外中心完成心脏心外科手术22 190例，其中阜外医院（北京）13 149例，阜外华中心血管病医院5332例，深圳阜外心血管病医院1455例，云南阜外心血管病医院2028例。阜外医院为全国各地患者提供了优质的医疗服务。

According to the Law on basic Medical Care and Health Promotion and the requirements of "the 14th five-year Plan" issued by the State Council, Fuwai Hospital has made great efforts to promote the establishment of "double centers" in construction. At present, it has formed a model of one national center and three regional sub-centers. Fuwai Hospital in Beijing serves as the national medical center, Fuwai Central China Cardiovascular Hospital, Fuwai Hospital in Shenzhen and Fuwai Yunnan Cardiovascular Hospital as regional medical centers, realizing the strategic layout of "dual centers".

Fuwai Hospital has carried out in-depth research on core technologies, focusing on solving long-term and overall medical problems affecting people's health. It is of great strategic significance to improve China s medical service system, lead the development of medical science and improve the overall medical service ability.

In 2022, 22,190 cases of cardiac surgery were performed in four Fuwai centers, including 13,149 cases in Fuwai Hospital (Beijing), 5332 cases in Fuwai Central China Cardiovascular Hospital, 1455 cases in Fuwai Hospital in Shenzhen and 2028 cases in Fuwai Yunnan Cardiovascular Hospital. Fuwai Hospital provides high-quality medical services for patients all over the country.

▶ 外科手术量及术后30日死亡率
Volume and 30-day mortality

2022年，阜外医院心血管外科手术共计13 149例，术后30日死亡率为0.49%，已连续14年低于1%，在世界各大心脏中心居于领先水平（图1-1）。

In 2022, a total of 13,149 cardiovascular surgeries were performed in Fuwai Hospital, with a 30-day postoperative mortality rate of 0.49%. The rate has been below 1% for 14 consecutive years, which is at a leading level among major cardiac centers around the world (Figure 1-1).

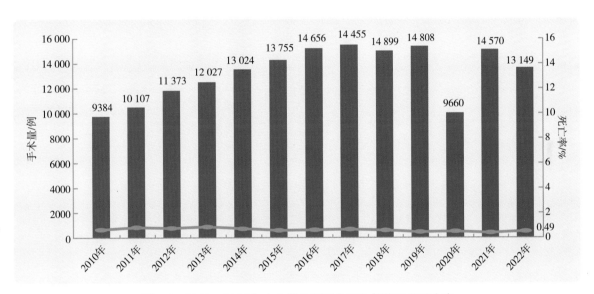

图1-1　2010—2022年心血管外科手术量及术后30日死亡率
Figure 1-1　Volume and 30-day mortality, 2010—2022

▶ 手术分类构成
Classification of surgery

阜外医院作为中国最大的心脏中心，医院收治患者的病因学分类基本反映了我国心血管外科疾病治疗谱。先天性心脏病和瓣膜病呈总体下降趋势，而主动脉外科手术、心脏移植等呈总体增加趋势（图1-2）。

As the largest heart center in China, Fuwai Hospital s classification of the causes of patients treated reflects the basic profile of cardiovascular surgical diseases in China. Congenital heart disease and valve disease have shown an overall decreasing trend, while surgeries for aortic diseases and heart transplantation have shown an overall increasing trend (Figure 1-2).

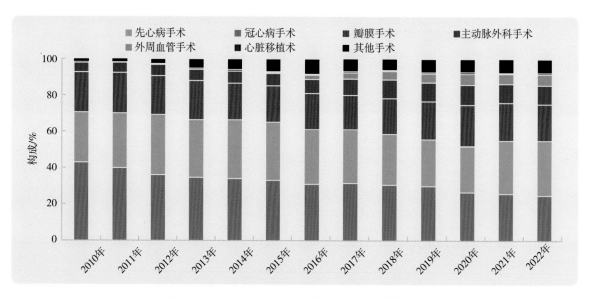

图1-2　2010—2022年心血管外科手术分类构成

Figure 1-2　Classification of surgery, 2010—2022

▶ 各术种手术死亡率
Mortality rate of each surgical category

阜外医院已连续多年做到不同种类的心血管外科手术30日死亡率均低于1%（图1-3），这体现了阜外医院在心血管外科手术的规范化管理、整体医疗质量的控制和疾病的综合救治水平均已达到世界先进水平。Fuwai hospital has maintained a 30-day mortality rate of less than 1% for various types of cardiovascular surgical procedures for many years, which reflects the standardized management of cardiovascular surgical procedures, the overall control of medical quality, and the comprehensive treatment levels for cardiovascular diseases of Fuwai hospital have reached world-class standards (Figure 1-3).

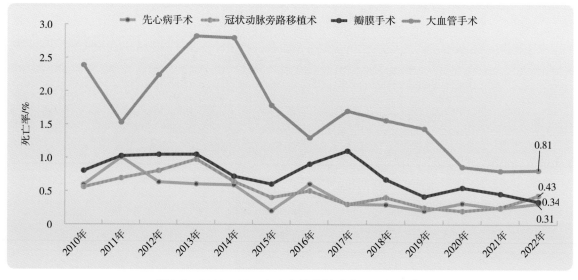

图1-3　2010—2022年心血管外科手术30日死亡率

Figure 1-3　Mortality rate in 30-day post-surgery of each surgical category, 2010—2022

▶ 各术种术后住院天数
Mortality rate of each surgical category

在外科、重症医学科、临床检验科、影像科、心脏康复中心等多学科共同努力和紧密配合下，阜外医院外科全术种的术后住院天数仍保持在平均9天以内，与去年基本持平（图1-4）。

Through the joint efforts and close cooperation of multiple department, such as surgery, intensive care medicine, clinical laboratory, imaging, and cardiac rehabilitation center, the postoperative hospital stay of all surgical procedures in our hospital remains within 9 days, which is basically the same as last year (Figure 1-4).

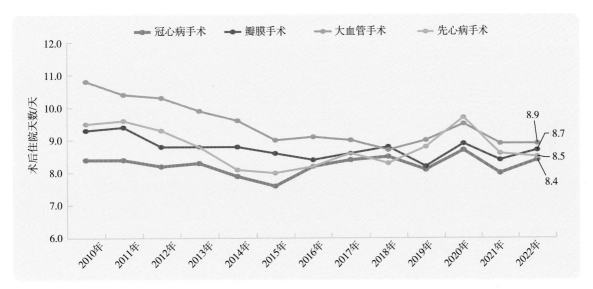

图1-4 2010—2022年外科手术后住院天数

Figure 1-4 Postoperative hospital stay, 2010—2022

▶ 急诊手术量及死亡率
Volume and mortality of emergency surgery

2022年，阜外医院急诊手术量已恢复至新型冠状病毒流行前水平。在新型冠状病毒感染的影响下，术前心肺功能不全导致急重症心血管病患者的急诊手术比例和术后死亡率保持在较低水平（图1-5）。

By the year 2022, the volume of emergency surgeries in Fuwai hospital has returned to the level before the outbreak of the COVID-19. Under the influence of COVID-19, there has been a slight increase in the proportion of emergency surgeries and postoperative mortality rates among critically cardiovascular disease patients with preoperative cardiopulmonary dysfunction compared to previous years (Figure 1-5).

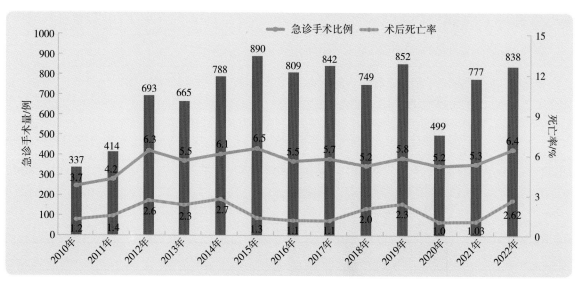

图1-5　2010—2022年术前心肺功能不全致急重症心血管病患者的急诊手术量和术后死亡率

Figure 1-5　Volume and mortality of emergency surgery, 2010—2022

▶ 手术患者的年龄分布
Age distribution of patients

60岁以上的老年人和40～60岁的中年人在总手术人群中占比过半（图1-6），体现了心血管病仍是我国中老年人最容易罹患的疾病之一。

People aged 60 and above, as well as those aged between 40 and 60, account for over half of the total number of surgeries (Figure 1-6), which reflects that cardiovascular disease remains one of the most common diseases among middle-aged and elderly people in China.

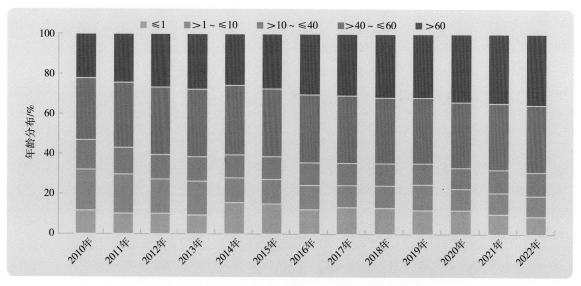

图1-6　2010—2022年心血管外科手术患者的年龄分布

Figure 1-6　Age distribution of patients, 2010—2022

► 先天性心脏病手术量及手术死亡率
Volume and mortality of congenital heart surgery

2022年，阜外医院共完成先天性心脏病手术3257例，死亡率仅为0.3%（图1–7）。

In 2022, the volume of congenital heart surgeries was 3257, with an extremely low mortality of 0.3% (Figure 1–7).

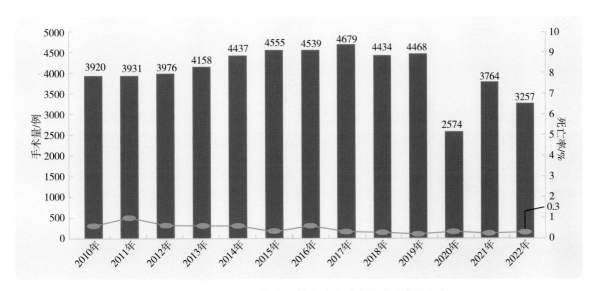

图1-7　2010—2022年先天性心脏病手术量及手术死亡率

Figure 1-7　Volume and mortality of congenital heart surgery, 2010—2022

二、先天性心脏病
Congenital heart diseases

► **危重复杂先心病手术数量**
Volume of critical and complex congenital heart surgery

阜外医院作为中国最大的先天性心脏病中心，肩负着收治全国范围内急、危重症和复杂畸形的先心病患儿。2020年起，危重复杂先心病患儿比例显著升高，2022年阜外医院共收治2666例复杂先心病患儿，占总收治患儿数的81.9%（图1-8）。

As the largest congenital heart disease center in China, Fuwai Hospital shoulders the responsibility of treating critically complex congenital heart disease patients from all over the country. Since 2020, the proportion of critically complex congenital heart disease patients has significantly increased. In 2022, our hospital treated a total of 2666 complex congenital heart disease patients, accounting for 81.9% of total admissions (Figure 1-8).

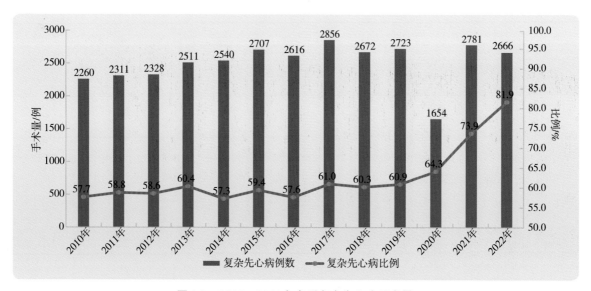

图1-8　2010—2022年危重复杂先心病手术量

Figure 1-8　Volume of critical and complex congenital heart surgery, 2010—2022

► 新生儿手术量及死亡率
Volume of congenital heart surgery for neonatal

"新生儿先心病绿色通道"和"新生儿产前产后一体化救治体系"是阜外医院小儿外科中心的特色诊疗，实现了新生儿从出生到院际间转运、围手术期监护、手术、术后康复及随访一体化管理。2022年阜外医院新生儿手术量较去年增加30%，手术死亡率仅为3.3%，仍与去年保持相同水平（图1-9）。

The "Green Channel for Neonatal Congenital Heart Disease" and "Integrated treatment system for newborns before and after birth" are distinctive feature of diagnosis and treatment in our Pediatric Surgery Center, which achieves integrated management of neonatal patients from birth to inter-hospital transfer, perioperative monitoring, surgery, postoperative recovery, and follow-up. In 2022, the number of neonatal surgeries in our hospital increased by 30% compared to last year, with a surgical mortality rate of only 3.3%, which remains at the same level as last year (Figure 1-9).

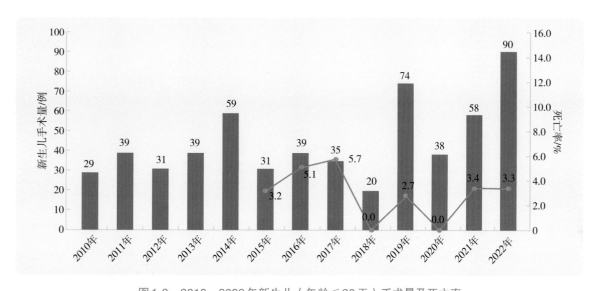

图1-9　2010—2022年新生儿（年龄≤28天）手术量及死亡率
Figure 1-9　Volume of congenital heart surgery for neonatal, 2010—2022

► 低体重患儿比例
Propotion of patients with low body weight

低龄、低体重是危重先心病患儿的重要临床特点。2022年阜外医院低体重患儿的比例达到5.6%，为近十年最高（图1-10）。

Low age and low body weight are important clinical characteristics of critically ill children with congenital heart disease. In 2022, the proportion of low body weight children in Fuwai Hospital reached 5.6%, the highest in nearly a decade (Figure 1-10).

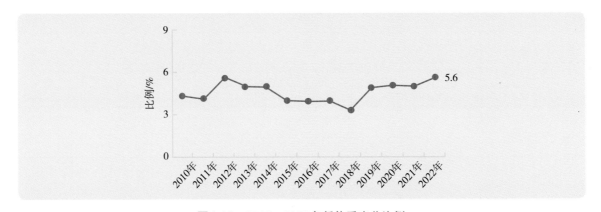

图 1-10 2010—2022 年低体重患儿比例

Figure 1-10 Propotion of neonatal with low body weight, 2010—2022

▶ **平均术后住院天数**
Average postoperative length of stay

优质、高效的医疗可以缩短患者的住院时间。阜外医院2022年先天性心脏病患儿的平均住院天数仅为8.5天（图1-11）。

High-quality and efficient medical care can shorten the hospitalization time. In 2022, the average length of stay for children with congenital heart disease in Fuwai hospital was only 8.5 days (Figure 1-11).

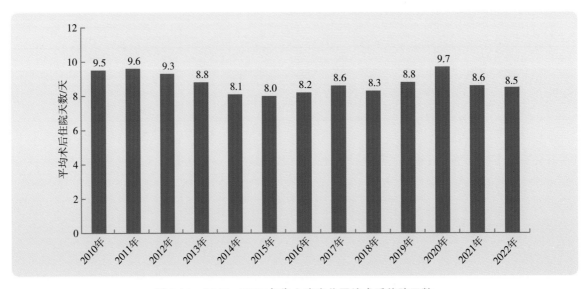

图 1-11 2010—2022 年先心病患儿平均术后住院天数

Figure 1-11 Average postoperative length of stay, 2010—2022

三、冠状动脉粥样硬化性心脏病
Coronary artery diseases

► **单纯冠状动脉旁路移植术（CABG）手术量和死亡率**
Volume and mortality of isolated coronary artery bypass grafting

2022年，冠状动脉旁路移植术手术量与往年基本持平，30日死亡率保持低水平。阜外医院共完成冠状动脉旁路移植术4529例，其中单纯冠状动脉旁路移植术3274例，30日死亡率已连续9年低于0.5%（图1-12）。

In 2022, the volume remains the same as in previous years and the 30-day mortality remains in very low level. 4529 patients underwent isolated or combined CABG at Fuwai Hospital, with 3274 cases of isolated CABG. The 30-day mortality has remained stable over the past 9 years at a level of less than 0.5% (Figure 1-12).

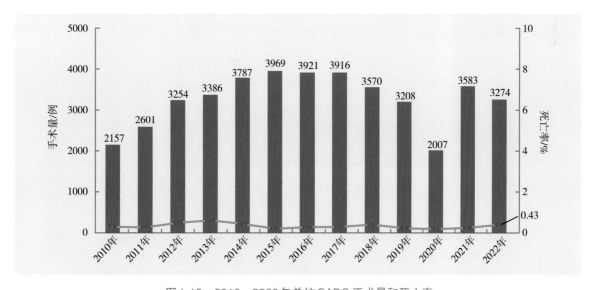

图1-12　2010—2022年单纯CABG手术量和死亡率

Figure 1-12　Volume and mortality of isolated coronary artery bypass grafting, 2010—2022

▶ 单纯CABG移植物构成情况
Usage of bypass conduits in cabg

阜外医院动脉桥的使用率维持在95%以上。我们根据患者个体情况优化治疗策略，常规开展双侧乳内动脉、桡动脉、全动脉化和"no-touch"获取大隐静脉技术，旨在为不同患者提供高质量、个性化的血运重建策略（图1-13）。

The use of left internal thoracic artery is over 95% for years at Fuwai. The surgical team of Fuwai Hospital intended to provide individualized optimal revascularization strategies for patients. Multiple approaches, such as bilateral internal thoracic artery, radial artery, total arterial grafts, "no touch" technique for great saphenous vein harvest, are also routinely performed at our institution (Figure 1-13).

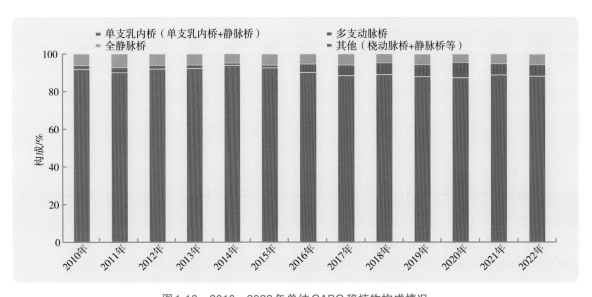

图1-13　2010—2022年单纯CABG移植物构成情况

Figure 1-13　Usage of bypass conduits in CABG, 2010—2022

▶ CABG同期瓣膜手术量和死亡率
Volume and mortality of cabg combined with valve surgery

阜外医院CABG同期瓣膜手术的患者占比逐年升高。尽管此类患者手术难度和复杂性显著增加，我院始终将30日死亡率控制在较低水平。2022年，我院共完成此类手术730例，30日死亡率仅为1.1%（图1-14）。

The volume of CABG combined with valve surgery increased in Fuwai hospital. Although coronary surgery simultaneously with valvular surgery increases complexity, the perioperative mortality for this combined surgery has stabilized at a low level. In 2022, we performed 730 cases, the 30-day mortality mortality rate was 1.1% (Figure 1-14).

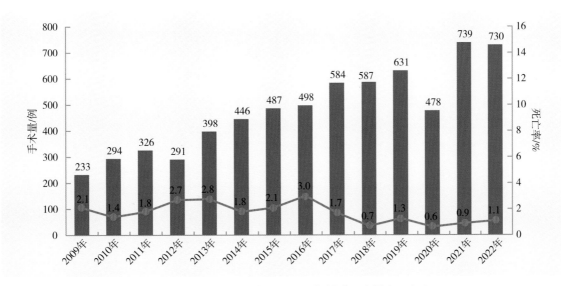

图1-14 2009—2022年CABG同期瓣膜手术量和死亡率

Figure 1-14 Volume and mortality of cabg combined with valve surgery, 2009—2022

▶ 室壁瘤修复手术量及死亡率
Volume and mortality of repairment of ventricular aneurysm

　　室壁瘤修复手术可让绝大多数患者远期获益，但是患者病情重，死亡率相对较高，这对术者及其医疗团队水平提出了更高的要求。2022年，阜外医院共完成室壁瘤手术95例，死亡率为4.2%（图1-15）。Ventricular aneurysm repairment could significantly improve the long-term outcomes for patients with coronary artery disease. However, the critical condition of this kinds of patients increased the risk of mortality. In 2022, we performed 95 cases of surgical repair for ventricular aneurysm, the perioperative mortality rate was 4.2% (Figure 1-15).

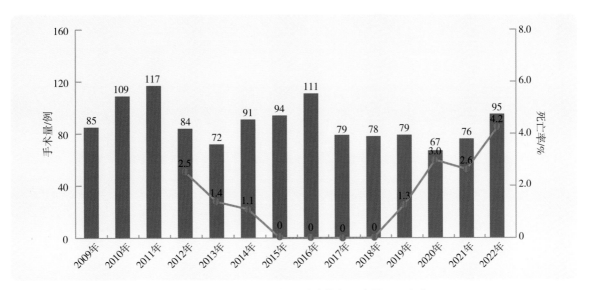

图1-15 2009—2022年室壁瘤修复手术量及死亡率

Figure 1-15 Volume and mortality of ventricular aneurysm repairment, 2009—2022

► CABG手术的平均术后住院天数
Post-operative length of stay of CABG

患者的康复依赖于高水平的手术技术、围手术期管理监护水平、康复管理水平。2022年，阜外医院CABG手术的平均术后住院天数为8.6天（图1-16），平均住院费用为137 831.15元，其中单纯CABG 8.1天（图1-17）。

The best cure included outstanding surgical technique, post-operative care and cardiac rehabilitation.The length of stay for all CABG and isolated CABG was 8.6 days and 8.1 days respectively in 2022, the awerage expenditure was 137 831.15RMB (Figure 1-16，Figure 1-17).

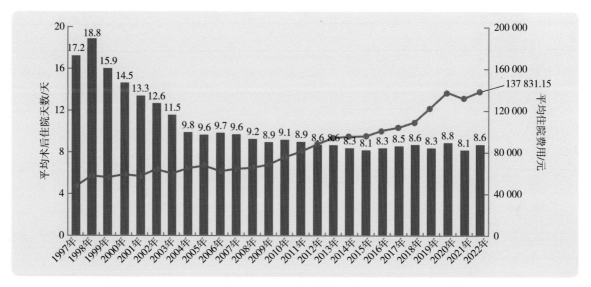

图1-16　1997—2022年CABG手术的平均术后住院天数和平均住院费用
Figure 1-16　Post-operative length of stay of CABG, 1997—2022

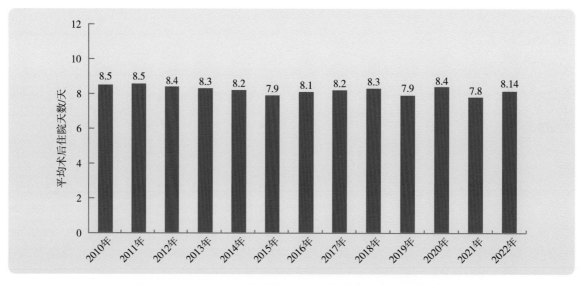

图1-17　2010—2022年单纯CABG手术的平均术后住院天数
Figure 1-17　Post-operative length of stay of isolated CABG, 2010—2022

四、心脏瓣膜病
Valvular heart diseases

▶ **心脏瓣膜手术量及死亡率**
Volume and mortality of cardiac valve surgery

　　阜外医院是我国最大的瓣膜外科中心。2022年，我院共完成心脏瓣膜手术4399例，30天死亡率仅为0.4%（图1-18）。

Fuwai Hospital is the largest cardiac valve surgery center in China. In 2022, 4399 patients received valvular operation at our institution with a 30-day mortality of 0.4% (Figure 1-18).

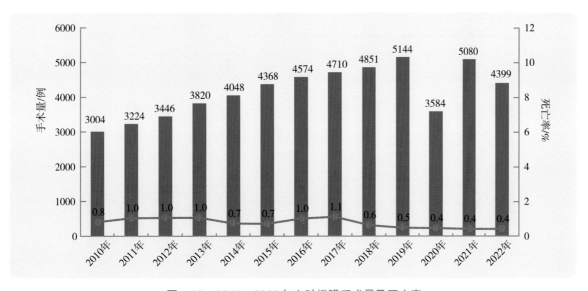

图1-18　2010—2022年心脏瓣膜手术量及死亡率
Figure 1-18　Volume and mortality of cardiac valve surgery, 2010—2022

► 心脏瓣膜手术病因构成
Etiologic distribution of cardiac valve surgery

瓣膜外科疾病病因占比变化显著，退行性变和先天性病因占比已超过风湿性病变，成为目前瓣膜病的主要病因，这也对瓣膜外科的治疗技术提出了新的要求（图1-19）。

The etiology of valve diseases changed significantly. Currently, degenerative valve disease and congenital valve disease has surpassed rheumatic valve disease, and became the major causes, which requested modern surgical techniques (Figure 1-19).

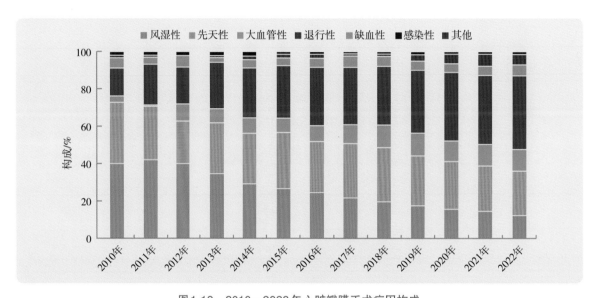

图1-19　2010—2022年心脏瓣膜手术病因构成

Figure 1-19　Etiologic distribution of cardiac valve surgery, 2010—2022

► 心脏瓣膜手术类型构成
Type of cardiac valve surgery

2022年，二尖瓣成形术再次占据瓣膜手术首位，主动脉瓣成形术占比也逐年升高，这是阜外医院瓣膜综合修复技术的体现（图1-20）。

In 2022, mitral valve repairment represented the major proportion of all valvar surgeries for the second time. The aortic valve repairment technique improved a lot as well. These data demonstrated the outstanding valve repairment technique at Fuwai (Figure 1-20).

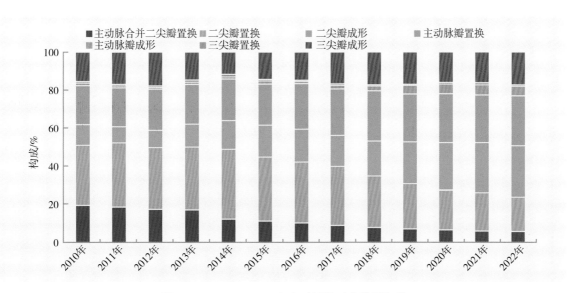

图1-20　2010—2022年心脏瓣膜手术类型构成

Figure 1-20　Type of cardiac valve surgery, 2010—2022

▶ **单纯二尖瓣置换手术量及死亡率**
Volume and mortality of isolated mitral valve replacement

阜外医院2022年共完成单纯二尖瓣置换术336例，30天死亡率仅为0.6%（图1-21）。

In 2022, we performed 336 cases of mitral valve replacement in Fuwai. The 30-day mortality was only 0.6% (Figure 1-21).

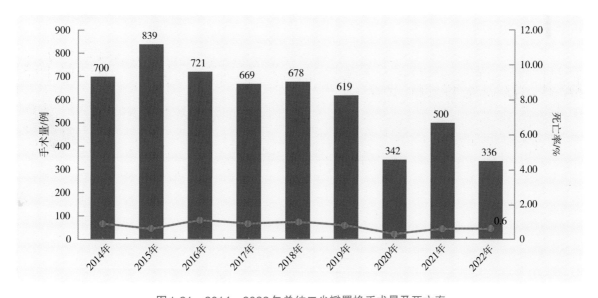

图1-21　2014—2022年单纯二尖瓣置换手术量及死亡率

Figure 1-21　Volume and mortality of isolated mitral valve replacement, 2014—2022

► **单纯二尖瓣关闭不全患者瓣膜成形与置换量**

Volume of valvuloplasty versus replacement for isolated mitral valve regurgitaion

瓣膜成形技术手段越来越多，修复成功率稳步提高。阜外医院外科团队开展全面、规范、优质的瓣膜成形术，疗效显著。2022年，我院共完成单纯二尖瓣关闭不全患者的二尖瓣成形术619例，占比达80.1%（图1-22）。

As our deep understanding of the structure and function of cardiac valves, the methods to repairing valves increased, with the improvement of repair rates. Fuwai Hospital can perform comprehensive, standardized and superior valve repairment procedures. In the year of 2022, 80.1% (619 cases) of all mitral valve regurgitation cases underwent surgical repairment procedures (Figure 1-22).

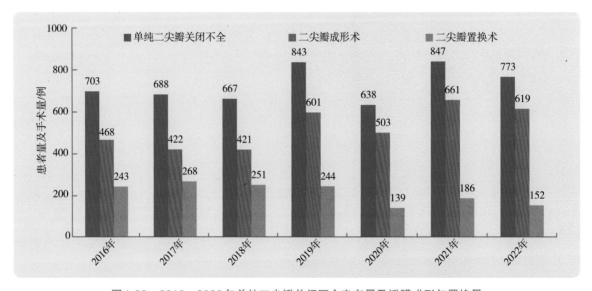

图1-22　2016—2022年单纯二尖瓣关闭不全患者量及瓣膜成形与置换量

Figure 1-22　Volume of valvuloplasty versus replacement for isolated mitral valve regurgitaion, 2016—2022

► **单纯主动脉瓣置换手术量及死亡率**

Volume and mortality of isolated aortic valve replacement

2022年，阜外医院共完成单纯主动脉瓣置换手术462例，30天死亡率为0（图1-23）。

In 2022, the volume of isolated aortic valve replacement in Fuwai was 462, and the 30-day mortality was 0 (Figure 1-23).

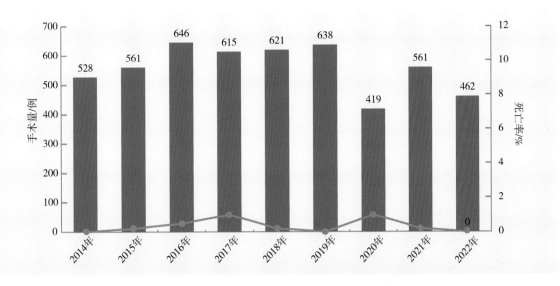

图 1-23　2014—2022 年单纯主动脉瓣置换手术量及死亡率

Figure 1-23　Volume and mortality of isolated aortic valve replacement, 2014—2022

▶ 心脏瓣膜手术术后平均住院天数
Post-operative length of stay of cardiac valve surgery

瓣膜手术的术后平均住院天数是重要的医疗质量评价指标。阜外医院心脏瓣膜手术术后平均住院天数为9天（图1-24）。

The post-operative length of stay is one critically important quality measure for valve surgery. The post-operative length of stay at Fuwai was only 9 days (Figure 1-24).

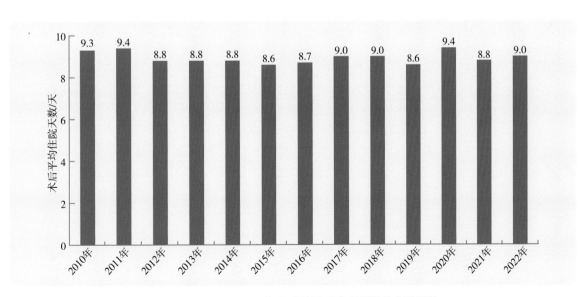

图 1-24　2010—2022 年心脏瓣膜手术术后平均住院天数

Figure 1-24　Post-operative length of stay of cardiac valve surgery, 2010—2022

五、主动脉疾病
Aortic diseases

▶ 主动脉外科手术量
Volume of aortic surgery

2022年，阜外医院共完成主动脉外科手术治疗1355例，主动脉腔内支架修复手术527例。本数据不包括小儿外科中心专家完成的小儿主动脉手术（图1-25）。

In 2022, there were 1355 open aortic surgery, and 527 endovascular aortic repairs. Our data do not include the aortic operations for infant and children performed at the Pediatric Cardiac Surgical Center (Figure 1-25).

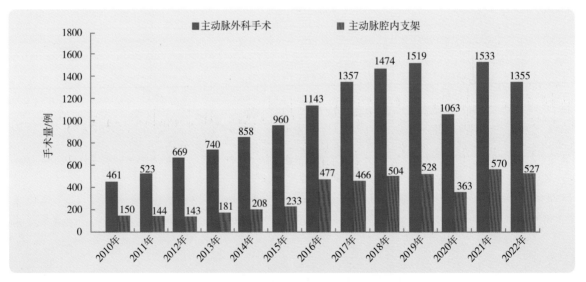

图1-25　2010—2022年主动脉外科手术量

Figure 1-25　Volume of aortic surgery, 2022

► **主动脉外科手术治疗部位构成**
Treatment region underwent aortic surgery

2022年，阜外医院主动脉外科手术中，主动脉弓部病变占36.2%，主动脉根部和升主动脉病变占31.4%，降主动脉病变占16.2%，腹主动脉病变占14.5%，胸腹主动脉病变占1.7%（图1-26）。

These figure shows the composition of open, endovascular, and hybrid aortic procedures at Fuwai Hospital over the past decade. In 2022, 31.4% of procedures were on the aortic root and ascending aorta, 36.2% were for aortic arch, 16.2% for descending aorta, 14.5% abdominal aorta, and 1.7% for thoracoabdominal aorta (Figure 1-26).

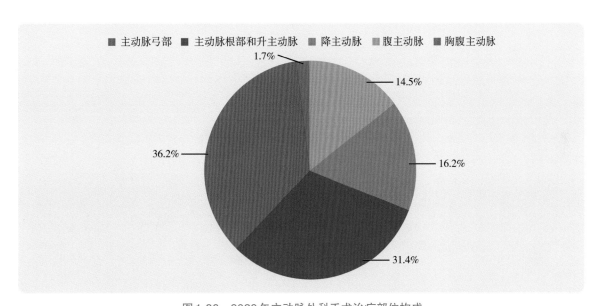

图1-26　2022年主动脉外科手术治疗部位构成

Figure 1-26　Treatment region underwent aortic surgery, 2010—2022

► **主动脉外科手术患者年龄**
Age distribution of aortic surgery

近十年来，接受主动脉外科、腔内和杂交手术的患者中，60岁以上患者比例呈现逐步增加的趋势（图1-27）。

In recent 10 years, the proportion of patients over 60 years of age who underwent open, endovascular, or hybrid aortic procedures at Fuwai Hospital increased significantly (Figure 1-27).

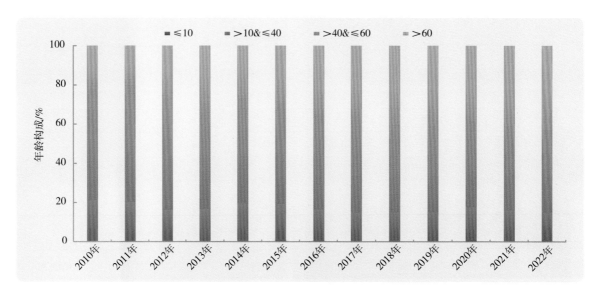

图1-27 2010—2022年主动脉外科手术患者年龄构成

Figure 1-27 Age distribution of aortic surgery, 2010—2022

▶ 大血管手术择期、急诊手术例数和死亡率
Volume and mortality of elective and emergency aortic surgery

主动脉急症常需要紧急手术，技术难度大，手术风险高。阜外医院集全院优势力量，从制度层面入手，建立了"胸痛中心"和"主动脉急诊绿色通道"，在主动脉急症患者的救治效率和救治成功率方面均已成为我国典范。2022年，我院血管外科完成急诊手术234例，术后30天死亡率仅为3.0%（图1-28）。Aortic emergencies, including acute aortic syndrome and aortic rupture, are usually life-threatening, sudden onset catastrophes of the aorta that present immense surgical technique challenges and have high associated risk. The Aortic Emergency Green Channel policy of Fuwai Hospital has been in place for several years and has helped ensure that the majority of emergent aortic patients are treated in an efficient manner. The hospital continues to have one of the highest technical success rates for emergent aortic operations in the world. In 2022, surgeons at the Vascular Surgery Center performed 234 emergent aortic surgeries, with 30-day mortality of 3.0% (Figure 1-28).

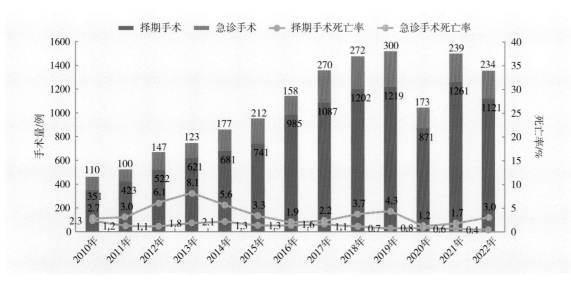

图1-28　2010—2022年大血管手术择期、急诊手术量和死亡率

Figure 1-28　Volume and mortality of elective and emergency aortic surgery, 2010—2022

► 主动脉夹层手术量和死亡率
Volume and mortality of surgical treatment for aortic dissection

我国高血压病患者的知晓率、治疗率、控制率偏低，因此，主动脉夹层发病率较高，对患者、家庭和社会造成了极大的负担。阜外医院常年为此类患者提供紧急手术，挽救生命。2022年，我院共完成主动脉夹层手术420例，术后30天死亡率仅为1.2%，创造历史最低死亡率（图1-29）。

The rates of awareness, treatment and control of hypertension in China were low, with the consequence of high prevalence of aortic dissection. We provide emergent surgery service for these patients. In 2022, we performed a total of 420 aortic procedures for aortic dissection with a 30-day postoperative mortality of 1.2%, which is the lowest mortality rate in Fuwai history (Figure 1-29).

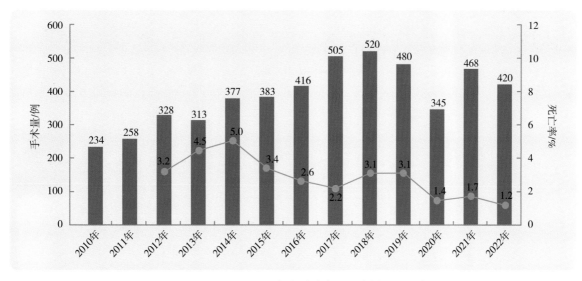

图1-29　2010—2022年主动脉夹层手术量和死亡率

Figure 1-29　Volume and mortality of surgical treatment for aortic dissection, 2010—2022

▶ David 手术量
Volume of David procedure

2022年，阜外医院共完成82例保留主动脉瓣的主动脉根部置换术（图1-30）。

In 2022, surgeons at the Vascular Surgery Center performed 82 David procedures (Figure 1-30).

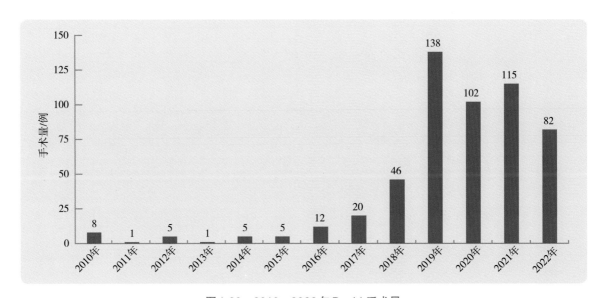

图1-30 2010—2022年David 手术量

Figure 1-30 Volume of David procedure, 2010—2022

▶ 主动脉微创腔内修补术
Minimally invasive intracavitary repair of aorta

2022年，阜外医院血管外科中心完成主动脉覆膜支架腔内修复术527例，我院已经将"烟囱"技术、"潜望镜"技术、"开窗"技术等新型辅助技术纳入日常诊疗常规，为主动脉病变，包括主动脉弓部病变的患者提供腔内修复治疗（图1-31）。

In 2022, surgeons at the Vascular Surgery Center performed 527 endovascular operations. The chimney, snorkel, and fenestration techniques were routinely used by us for the treatment of patients with aortic (including aortic arch) diseases (Figure 1-31).

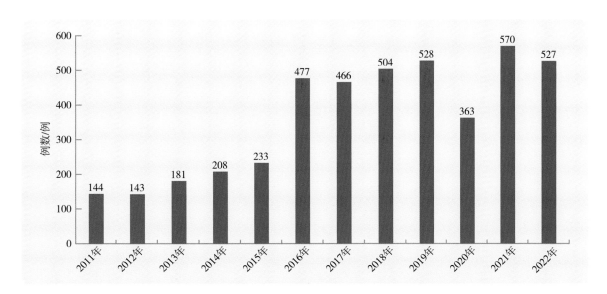

图1-31　2011—2022年主动脉微创腔内修补术例数

Figure 1-31　Volume of minimally invasive intracavitary repair of aorta, 2011—2022

► **主动脉外科手术患者术后平均住院天数和平均住院费用**
Cost and post-operative length of stay of aortic surgery

阜外医院主动脉外科手术患者的术后平均住院天数仅为8.9天，体现了较高的外科治疗和术后监护、康复管理水平（图1-32）。

The post-operative length of stay after aortic procedures was only 8.9 days (Figure 1-32).

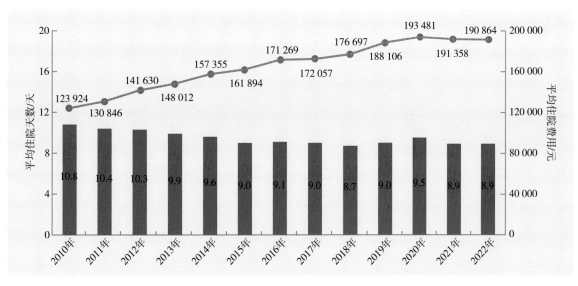

图1-32　2010—2022年主动脉外科手术患者术后平均住院天数和平均住院费用

Figure 1-32　Cost and post-operative length of stay of aortic surgery, 2010—2022

▶ 周围血管疾病手术量
Volume of peripheral vascular surgery

　　2015年底，阜外医院增设外科血管疾病治疗团队，主要以外科动脉、静脉疾病的介入和外科治疗作为主攻方向。2022年，我院共实施1506例外科血管开放和介入手术（图1-33）。

A dedicated peripheral vascular ward was established at Fuwai Hospital in November 2015. Ward staff include Team A vascular surgeons and Team B interventional cardiologists. In 2022, the two teams performed 1506 interventional and open procedures on patients with peripheral vascular diseases (Figure 1-33).

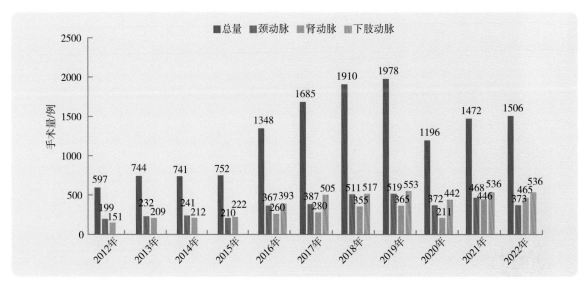

图1-33　2012—2022年周围血管疾病手术量

Figure 1-33　Volume of peripheral vascular surgery, 2012—2022

▶ 心脏移植手术量和死亡率
Volume and mortality of heart transplantation

　　2022年，阜外医院共完成115例心脏移植手术，移植后患者30天死亡率仅为0.9%（图1-34）。我院自开展心脏移植手术以来，累计完成心脏移植手术1210例，是我国心脏移植体量最大的心脏外科中心。长期随访显示，我院心脏移植术后患者1年生存率为94.1%，5年生存率为88.4%，10年生存率为78.1%，均明显高于国际心肺移植协会（ISHLT）统计的同期生存率。

At Fuwai Hospital, we performed 115 cases of heart transplantation in 2022, and the 30-day mortality was only 0.9% (Figure 1-34). 1210 patients have undergone heart transplantation at Fuwai Hospital, As the largest heart transplantation center in China, the 1-year, 5-year and 10-year survival rates were 94.1%, 88.4% and 78.1%, respectively, which were significantly higher than the report by ISHLT.

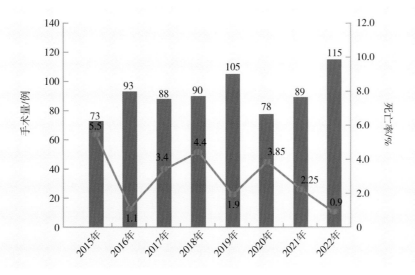

图 1-34　2015—2022 年心脏移植手术量和死亡率

Figure 1-34　Volume and mortality of heart transplantation, 2015—2022

▶ ECMO 辅助治疗情况
Usage of ECMO

　　在阜外医院，ECMO 广泛应用于急性心源性休克患者的救治。医生在成人和小儿心脏疾病的 ECMO 应用中都积累了极为丰富的经验。ECMO+IABP 已成为短期心肺辅助的常规应用，2022 年总计实施 ECMO 辅助治疗 42 例，并且取得良好效果（图 1-35 ）。

ECMO is widely used at Fuwai Hospital for patients with acute cardiogenic shock, for both children and adults. ECMO+IABP is routinely used for short-term ventricular assistance, 42 cases of ECMO were performed in 2022. Both applications have achieved excellent outcomes (Figure 1-35).

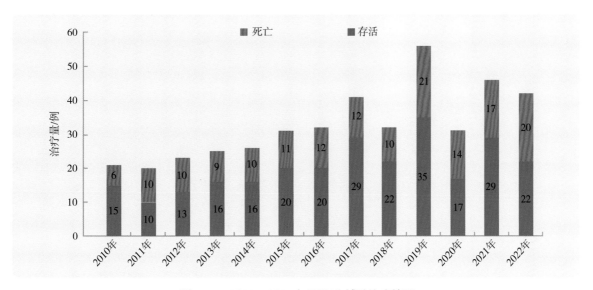

图 1-35　2010—2022 年 ECMO 辅助治疗情况

Figure 1-35　Usage of ECMO, 2010—2022

► **左室辅助手术量**
Volume of left ventricular assist device (LVAD)

　　左心室辅助装置治疗终末期心脏衰竭患者围手术期生存率96%，1年生存率96%，2年生存率 92%，3年生存率89%，携带装置生存时间最长已近5年。 2022年，LVAD手术量为27例，较往年显著增加（图1-36）。

The perioperative survival rate of end-stage heart failure patients with left ventricular assist device was 96%, the 1-year survival rate was 96%, the 2-year survival rate was 92%, the 3-year survival rate was 89%, and the longest survival time with device was 5 years. In 2022, the volume of LVAD was 27, which was significantly higher than that in previous years (Figure 1-36).

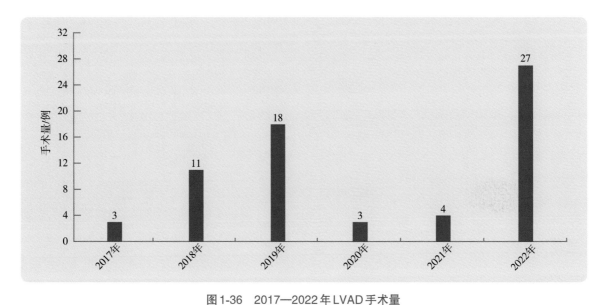

图 1-36　2017—2022 年 LVAD 手术量

Figure 1-36　Volume of left ventricular assist Device (LVAD), 2017—2022

六、其他疾病
Others

▶ 阜外 LVAD 手术总体概况
Overview of LVAD in fuwai

2017年6月至2023年3月，阜外医院及分院累计开展LVAD植入术102例，术前患者以INTER-MACS 2级为主，主要病因为扩张性心肌病和缺血性心肌病（图1-37）。

102 cases of LVAD implantation were performed in Fuwai hospital and three sub-centers. Preoperative patients were mainly INTERMACS grade 2, due to dilated cardiomyopathy and ischemic cardiomyopathy (Figure 1-37).

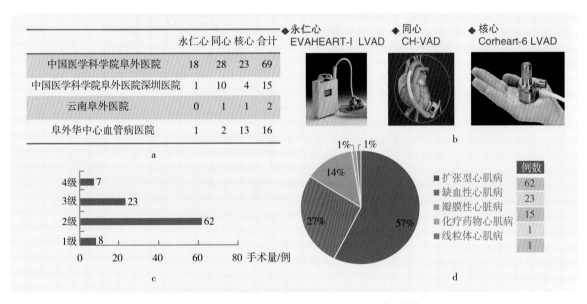

图1-37　2017年6月至2023年3月LVAD手术总体概况
注：a. LVAD手术量；b. LVAD类型；c. 术前分级；d. 病因学分析。
Figure 1-37　Overview of LVAD，2017—2023
a. Volume of LVAD; b. Type of LVAD; c. Preoperative classification; d. Pathological analysis.

► 杂交房颤射频消融手术量
Hybrid ablation for atrial fibrillation

阜外医院外科团队联合心律失常团队自2014年开展内外科复合消融手术，截至2022年，共完成复合消融手术105例，完成胸腔镜下心外膜消融手术195例（图1-38）。对于左房明显增大的难治性房颤患者，采用外科同期联合介入消融的治疗方式，介入强化消融或修饰消融可增加消融线路的透壁性。

Since 2014, the surgical team and the arrhythmia team of Fuwai Hospital have been carrying out hybrid ablation, and by 2022, 105 cases of hybrid ablation have been completed and 195 cases of thoracoscopy-assisted epicardial ablation (Figure 1-38). For patients with refractory atrial fibrillation and significantly enlarged left atrium, simultaneous surgical ablation combined with catheter ablation can increase the transmurality of ablation lesion set.

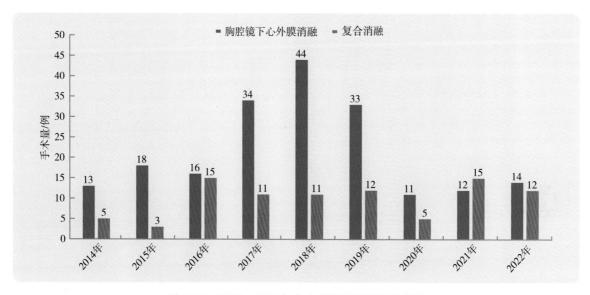

图1-38　2014—2022年杂交房颤射频消融手术量

Figure 1-38　Volume of hybrid ablation for atrial fibrillation, 2014—2022

► 肺栓塞的外科治疗
Surgical treatment for chronic thromboembolic pulmonary hypertension

阜外医院1997—2022年共开展肺动脉内膜剥脱术（PEA）298例。2015—2022年共完成193例PEA手术（图1-39），手术疗效达到国际领先水平。并在国内率先开展杂交技术（肺动脉内膜剥脱＋肺动脉球囊扩张术）治疗慢性血栓栓塞性肺动脉高压，成为开展此类治疗方案的全球最大中心之一。

From 1997 to 2022, a total of 298 cases of pulmonary endarterectomy (PEA) had been accomplished at Fuwai Hospital. In the last 8 years, 193 undertook PEA(Figure 1-39), which ranks the top in the world. Meanwhile, our center firstly carried out pulmonary endarterectomy + sequential pulmonary balloon angiography hybrid therapy strategy as the treatment of chronic thromboembolic pulmonary hypertension in mainland China，which is one of the largest centers in the world.

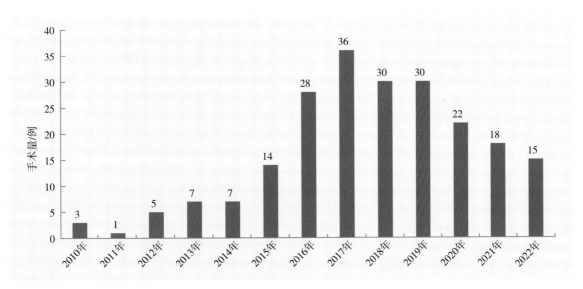

图1-39　2010—2022年EPA手术量

Figure 1-39　Volume of EPA, 2010—2022

► 微创心脏外科手术量
Volame of minimally invasive cardiac surgery

微创技术包括部分胸骨切口、右侧腋下小切口、胸骨旁切口、胸腔镜手术等，是减少患者手术创伤的重要技术手段，也是心脏外科的重点发展方向。2022年，阜外医院共完成微创心脏外科手术1404例（图1-40）。

The Fuwai surgical team is devoted to reducing surgical trauma for patients by using minimally invasive surgical techniques. The volume of these techniques, which include limited sternotomy, right subaxillary minithoractomy, and the parasternal approach, has steadily increased to 1404 in the year of 2022(Figure 1-40).

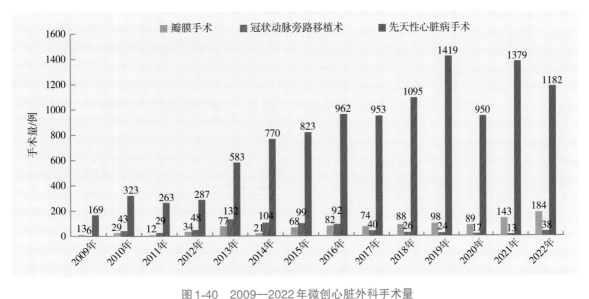

图1-40　2009—2022年微创心脏外科手术量

Figure 1-40　Volume of minimally invasive cardiac surgery , 2009—2022

▶ 胸腔镜手术量
Volume of thoracoscopic cardiac surgery

　　阜外医院常规开展胸腔镜系列手术，涵盖先天性心脏病矫治术、瓣膜成形置换和微创搭桥等。我院还针对阵发或持续性房颤患者开展全胸腔镜下心脏射频改良"迷宫"手术或联合心内膜消融的杂交射频消融手术，为难治性心房颤动患者带来新希望。2022年，我院共开展胸腔镜手术200例（图1-41）。

Video thoracoscope-assisted cardiac surgeries are routinely performed at Fuwai Hospital for congenital heart disease, cardiac valve repair or replacement, and minimally invasive coronary artery bypass surgeries. Favorable outcomes were achieved for persistent or concomitant atrial fibrillation by using hybrid thoracoscopic and catheter ablation(Figure 1-41).

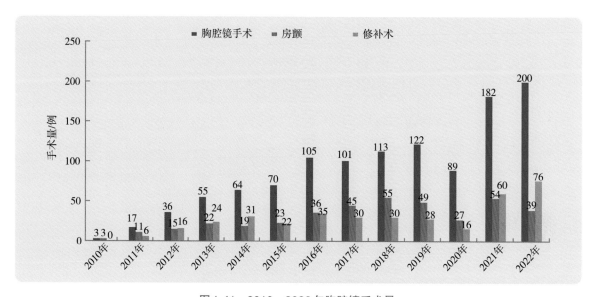

图1-41　2010—2022年胸腔镜手术量

Figure 1-41　Volume of thoracoscopic cardiac surgery, 2010—2022

▶ 经导管主动脉瓣植入术手术量
Volume of transcatheter aortic valve implantation (TAVI)

　　2012年9月，中国第一例国产经导管主动脉瓣在中国医学科学院阜外医院植入成功。阜外医院也首先开展了我国第一个TAVI临床试验。2014年7月，阜外医院外科团队运用我国自主研发的J-ValveTM瓣膜，在国内率先开展了经心尖入路的TAVI手术，不同于国际上TAVI技术仅用于主动脉瓣狭窄患者，阜外医院外科团队还在国际上首次为单纯主动脉瓣关闭不全患者成功实施了介入瓣膜的植入。2022年，我院共完成TAVI手术261例（图1-42）。

In September 2012, the first transcatheter aortic valve implantation (TAVI) procedure with a domestic valve was successfully performed. Fuwai Hospital has been committed to promoting the first clinical trial for TAVI in China. In July 2014, the Fuwai surgical team pioneered the use of the domestically-produced J-ValveTM to perform transapical aortic valve implantation. Because of the unique design of J-ValveTM, our team was the first in the world to successfully apply the TAVI technique on a patient with aortic insufficiency alone. In 2022, 261 patients with aortic valve disease successfully received this minimally invasive procedure(Figure 1-42).

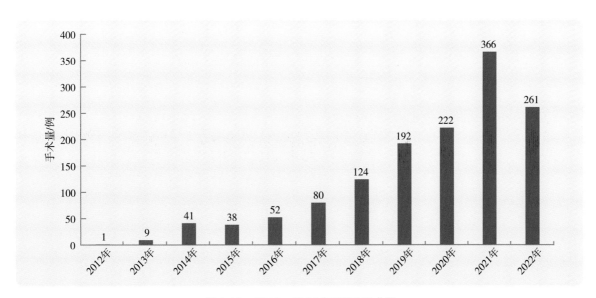

图1-42　2012—2022年TAVI手术量

Figure 1-42　Volume of TAVI, 2012—2022

OUTCOMES 2022

特色医疗
——
FEATURE
MEDICAL CARE

一、成人外科中心
Adult heart diseases

国内首例儿童植入式左心室辅助装置植入
The first case of LVAD implantation in children in China

　　14岁患儿，右心室双出口矫治术后13年，左室流出道重度狭窄，EF 16%，LVEDD 72mm，气管插管呼吸机辅助通气。胡盛寿院长亲自督导并主刀，集成人中心和小儿中心优势力量，积极救治患儿。术中植入Corheart 6 植入式左心室辅助装置+Konno术，手术顺利。术后3个月，患者心功能完全恢复，EF 60%，LVEDD 36mm，撤除装置（图2-1）。

Child, 14 years old, 13 years after surgery for double outlet of right ventricle, left ventricular outflow tract severe stenosis, EF 16%, LVEDD 72mm, tracheal intubation with ventilator-assisted ventilation. Corheart 6 implantable left ventricular assist device+Konno was implanted and the operation was successful. Three months after operation, the heart function of the patient recovered completely, EF 60%, LVEDD 36mm, removed the device (Figure 2-1).

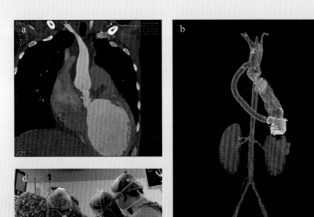
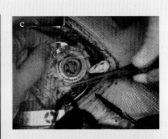
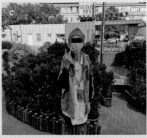

图2-1　国内首例儿童植入式左心室辅助装置

注：a. 术前影像；b. 术后3D重建；c. 术中影像；d. 术中照片；e. 患儿康复出院。

Figure 2-1　The first case of LVAD implantation in children in China

a. Preoperative Image; b. Postoperative 3d Reconstruction; c. Intraoperative Imaging Data; d. Intraoperative Photos;e. The child recovered and was discharged from hospital.

复合消融手术治疗难治性长程持续性房颤，术后1年维持窦性心律
Combined ablation for refractory long-period persistent atrial fibrillation and maintenance of sinus rhythm 1 year after operation.

　　63岁男性患者，BMI 37 kg/m²，心房颤动病史10年，转为持续性房颤4年，左房前后径62mm。心外科郑哲教授团队及心内科姚焰教授团队为患者行同期复合双房消融手术。外科消融后转为窦性心律，为患者获得更好的远期结果，外科消融后进行心内膜电生理标测及导管消融，对残余电位进行补充消融。术后1年，7天动态心电监测显示患者为窦性心律完全消除房颤（图2-2）。

A 63-year-old male patient, BMI 37 kg/m², with a history of 10 years of atrial fibrillation, converted to persistent atrial fibrillation for 4 years, and the left atrium anterior-posterior diameter was 62mm. Professor Zheng Zhe of cardiac surgical department and Professor Yao Yan of cardiology department performed combined biatrial ablation for the patients. After surgical ablation, ECG showed sinus rhythm. Cardiological team conducted endocardial electrophysiological mapping and catheter ablation to ablate the residual potential. One year after operation, 7-day ambulatory ECG monitoring showed sinus rhythm (Figure 2-2).

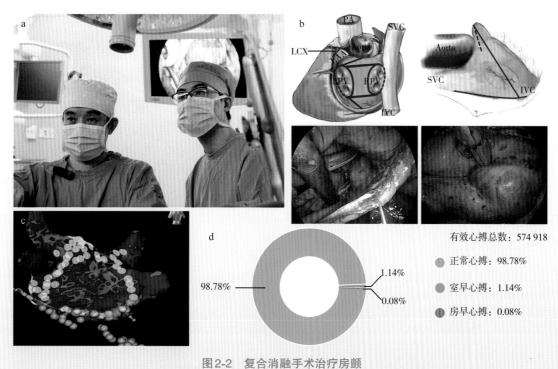

图2-2　复合消融手术治疗房颤
注：a. 手术医生；b. 手术模式图；c. 术中规划；d. 术后动态心电监测。
Figure 2-2　Combined ablation for atrial fibrillation
　　a. Intraoperative imaging data; b. Operation diagram; c. Intraoperative mapping; d. The operation completely eliminated atrial fibrillation.

全胸腔镜下改良扩大Morrow治疗梗阻性肥厚型心肌病
Thoracoscopic modified extended Morrow in the treatment of obstructive hypertrophic cardiomyopathy.

2021年5月至2022年10月，阜外医院共开展21例全胸腔镜下改良扩大Morrow手术（图2-3 a～f），患者平均年龄41.5岁，最年轻患者16岁，最年长患者65岁。全部手术无手术死亡和严重并发症，术后左心室流出道压差和室间隔厚度较术前显著降低（图2-3 g）。

From May 2021 to October 2022, Fuwai Hospital performed 21 cases of thoracoscopic modified extended Morrow surgery (Figure 2-3 a ~ f). The average age of the patients was 41.5 years old, the youngest patient was 16 years old, and the oldest patient was 65 years old. There was no operative death and serious complications. The left ventricular outflow tract pressure gradient and the thickness of interventricular septum decreased significantly after operation (Figure 2-3 g).

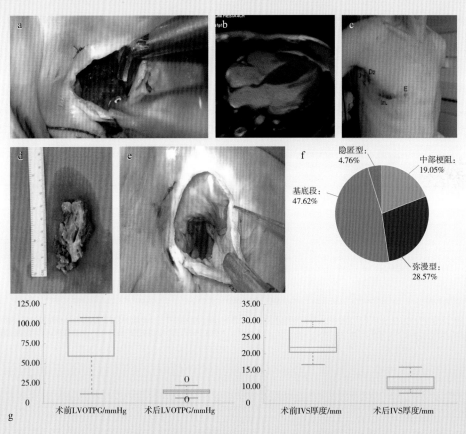

图2-3　全胸腔镜下改良扩大 Morrow 手术

注：a. 术前胸腔镜下可见流出道梗阻严重；b. 术前影像提示流出道严重梗阻；c. 手术微创切口；d. 手术标本；e. 术后流出道梗阻消除；f. 梗阻类型；g. 左心室流出道压差和室间隔厚度术前术后对比；LVOT，左心室流出道；IVS，室间隔。

Figure 2-3　Thoracoscopic modified extended Morrow

a. Severe obstruction of outflow tract could be seen under thoracoscope before operation；b. Preoperative imaging showed severe obstruction of the outflow tract；c. Small incision；d. Surgical specimens；e. The obstruction of outflow tract was eliminated after operation；f. Type of obstruction；g. Comparison of left ventricular outflow tract pressure gradient and interventricular septum thickness before and after operation；LVOT, left ventricular outflow tract；IVS, interventricular septum.

主动脉弓部一体式三分支覆膜支架系统技术的临床应用
Concave Supra-arch branched stent-graft system

该系统简化了主动脉弓部手术重建步骤和方式，有效缩短了手术时间，为广大医患提供了一种更简便的全腔内弓部病变微创修复方案，实现了主动脉弓部病变腔内治疗的突破。

与国际同类产品相比，我国具有完全自主知识产权的CS主动脉弓部分支支架系统具有以下优势：①无须定制，有效减少了术前等待时间和手术花费；②内漏风险小；③独特的凹槽设计实现了在隔绝病变的同时确保分支血供，避免术中脑部缺血，降低了卒中风险（图2-4a）。

The system simplifies the steps and methods of surgical reconstruction of aortic arch, effectively shortens the operation time, provides a more convenient minimally invasive repair scheme for doctors and patients, and realizes a breakthrough in endovascular treatment of aortic arch lesions. Compared with similar international products, China s completely independent intellectual property rights of CS aortic arch branch stent system has the following advantages: 1) no customization, which effectively reduces the preoperative waiting time and operation cost; 2) low risk of internal leakage; 3) the unique groove design realizes the protection of branch blood supply while isolating lesions, avoids cerebral ischemia during operation, and reduces the risk of stroke（Figure 2-4a）.

● **疑难病例：2023年1月完成阜外医院首例人体内植入术**
The first case of implantation in Fuwai hospital was completed in January 2023

51岁男性患者，检查发现弓部动脉瘤5年余（最大径：5.12cm），CTA提示主动脉弓部瘤累及Z1和Z2区，且邻近无名开口，需进行弓上三分支重建来保证双上肢、脑部的供血。因患者拒绝开放手术治疗，遂采用CS主动脉弓部分支重建系统行主动脉弓部三分支腔内修复手术。手术主体时间仅55分钟，总体手术时间130分钟，微创保留弓部三分支动脉血供，手术时间及费用均远低于传统外科治疗，术后患者恢复良好（图2-4 b～e）。

Male, 51 years old. Arch aneurysm, more than 5 years (maximum diameter: 5.12cm). CTA suggested that the aneurysm of the aortic arch involved Z1 and Z2 areas and was adjacent to the innominate orifice. Three branches of the supra arch should be reconstructed to ensure the blood supply to both upper limbs and brain. The patient refused open surgery, so endovascular repair of three branches of aortic arch was performed with CS partial aortic arch reconstruction system. The main time of the operation was only 55 minutes, and the overall operation time was 130 minutes. Minimally invasive preservation of the blood supply of the three branches of the arch artery, the operation time and cost were far lower than the traditional surgical treatment, and the patients recovered well after operation（Figure 2-4 b ~ e）。

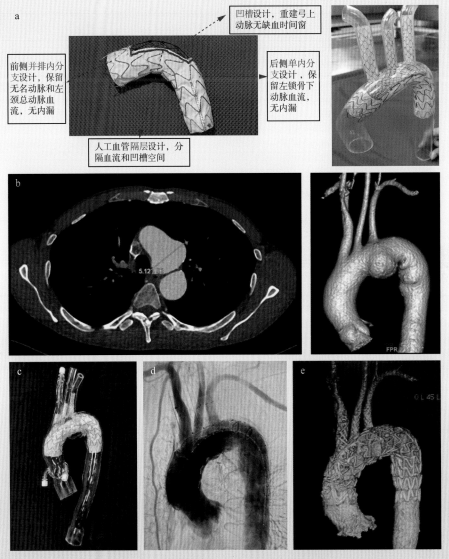

图 2-4　主动脉弓部一体式三分支覆膜支架

注：a. 主动脉弓部一体式三分支覆膜支架；b. 阜外首例主动脉弓部一体式三分支覆膜支架植入术术前主动脉CT；c. 术前3D打印患者主动脉模型并模拟体外植入；d. 术后造影；e. 术后一周复查主动脉CT。

Figure 2-4　Concave Supra-arch branched stent-graft system

a. Concave Supra-arch branched stent-graft system; b. Preoperative aortic CT; c. preoperative 3D printing of simulation of in vitro implantationpatient s aortic model; d. postoperative angiographic image; e. aortic CT is examined one week after operation.

设计研发针对胸腹主动脉疾病的定制多分支支架系统
Customized multi-branch stent graft system for thoracic and abdominal aortic diseases

该系统为个体化定制，采用微创手段实现内脏区多分支重建，有望打破进口支架的技术壁垒，减少患者的住院费用（图2-5）。

Individualized customization, the use of minimally invasive way to achieve multi-branch reconstruction of the visceral area is expected to break the technical barriers of imported stents and reduce the hospitalization costs (Figure 2-5).

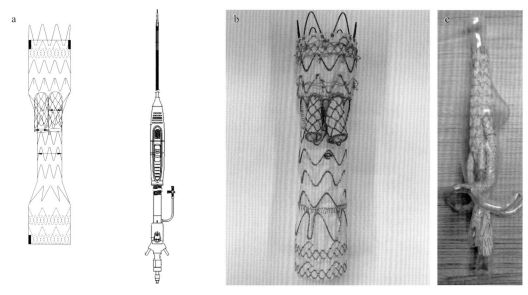

图2-5　个体化定制多分支支架系统
注：a. 支架设计图；b. 个体化多分支支架；c. 3D打印主动脉模型并模拟体外植入。
Figure 2-5　Customized multi-branch stent graft system
a. Stent design; b. Customized multi-branch stent; c. 3D printing of aortic model and simulation of in vitro implantation.

● **疑难病例：2021年1月完成全国首例人体内植入术**

68岁男性患者，2年前体检时发现胸腹主动脉瘤（6cm），4个月前出现胸背部疼痛，身体状况难以承受开放手术的巨大创伤，CTA检查提示：Crawford I型胸腹主动脉瘤，瘤体最大径约7cm，瘤体累及腹腔干、肠系膜上动脉、双肾动脉。在3D打印技术辅助下行定制胸腹主动脉四分支覆膜支架。手术主体时间仅53分钟，总体手术时间90分钟，微创保留内脏动脉血供，手术时间及费用均远远低于传统外科治疗，术后患者恢复良好（图2-6）。

A 68-year-old male was found with a thoraco-abdominal aortic aneurysm (TAAA, 6cm) during physical examination 2 years ago. 4 months later, he developed chest and back pain. CTA indicated a Crawford I TAAA with maximum diameter of 7cm. Four-branch stent graft for thoraco-abdominal aortic anueysm was customized with the help of 3D printing technology. The main operation time was only 53 minutes, the overall operation time was 90 minutes. The operation time and cost were far lower than traditional surgical treatment. All visceral arteries were preserved by endovascular technique (Figure 2-6).

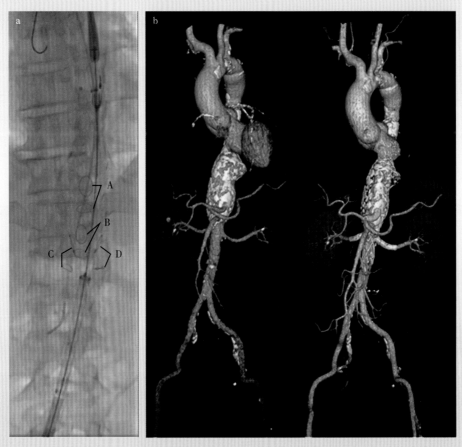

图2-6 国内首例定制胸腹主动脉四分支覆膜支架植入术

注：a. 术中造影；b. 3D重建胸腹主动脉。

Figure 2-6 The first four-branch stent graft implantation for thoraco-abdominal aortic aneurysm in China

a. Intraoperative angiography; b. 3D reconstruction of thoracic and abdominal aorta.

三、结构性心脏病中心
Structural heart diseases

▶ **经导管二尖瓣缘对缘修复技术（MitraClip）手术量居全国第一**
Volume of MitraClip ranks first in China

　　MitraClip是世界范围内使用最广泛的经导管二尖瓣介入器械，是我国目前唯一被批准的器械。2021年1月6日，阜外医院结构团队完成了MitraClip上市后第一例手术（图2-7）。目前，阜外医院结构团队是完成MitraClip手术最早、手术量最大的团队，也是国内唯一的带教团队。阜外技术升级："弯道超车"实现单纯经胸超声引导下MitraClip手术，保护患者、保护医生、降低医疗资源依赖程度，实现了极重度二尖瓣关闭不全患者床旁治疗。

MitraClip is the most widely used transcatheter mitral interventional instrument in the world, and it is the only approved instrument in China at present. On January 6, 2021, the structural team of Fuwai Hospital completed the first operation after MitraClip launching（Figure 2-7）. At present, Fuwai structure team is the first and largest team to complete Mitraclip. Fuwai Hospital Simple transthoracic ultrasound guided Mitraclip surgery could protect both patients and doctors, reduced dependence on medical resources and treated patients with extremely severe mitral regurgitation.

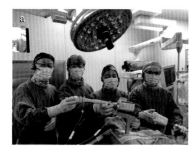 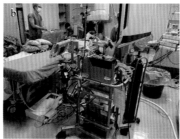 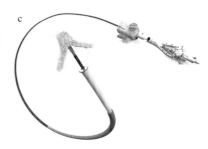

图2-7　MitraClip手术
注：a. 首例MitraClip手术；b. 术中影像资料；c. MitraClip。
Figure 2-7　MitraClip
a. The first MitraClip operation; b. Intraoperative imaging data; c. MitraClip.

四、小儿心脏中心
Congenital heart diseases

LVAD 治疗儿童终末期心力衰竭
LVAD in the treatment of end-stage heart failure in children

2022年，阜外医院完成国内首例儿童LVAD植入手术，总计完成3例LVAD植入术，LVAD相容性优异，疗效良好。

In 2022, Fuwai Hospital completed the first case of LVAD implantation in children, and a total of 3 cases of LVAD implantation were performed. LVAD achieved satisfactory compatibility and excellent therapeutic effect.

2022年6月
国内首例儿童LVAD植入

2022年8月
国内第二例儿童LVAD植入

2022年9月
国内首例儿童LVAD BTR撤泵

	性别	年龄	术前诊断	INTER MACS 分级	手术	支持时间/天	结局
1	男	14	右室双出口矫治术后左室流出道狭窄	2	Konno+VAD植入	98	撤除血泵
2	男	13	心肌致密化不全	2	VAD植入	256	继续携带
3	男	14	冠状动脉起源异常	2	VAD植入	20	继续携带

儿童长期携带微型磁悬浮心室辅助装置：良好相容性和有效性

图2-8 左心辅助装置治疗儿童终末心力衰竭

Figure 2-8 LVAD in the treatment of end-stage heart failure in children

肺动脉环缩+三腔起搏联合对抗小儿顽固性心力衰竭
Pulmonary artery banding combined with three-chamber pacemaker against heart failure in children

3月龄男性患儿，诊断为扩张性心肌病合并完全性左束支传导阻滞；左室EF 20%，左室舒张末期容积147ml；进行外科肺动脉环缩术抗心衰+CRT-P置入同步化治疗（图2-9）。

A 3-month-old male child was diagnosed as dilated cardiomyopathy with complete left bundle branch block; left ventricular EF was 20%, left ventricular end-diastolic volume was 147ml; pulmonary artery banding for heart failure plus CRT-P implantation synchronization therapy (Figure 2-9).

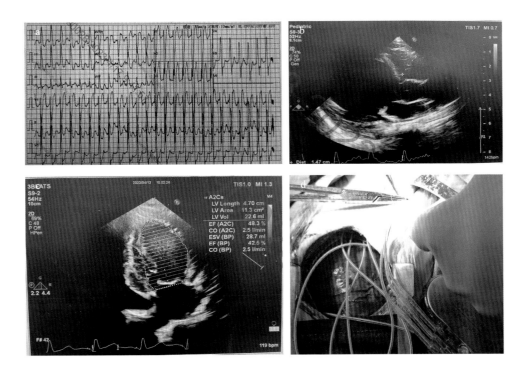

图2-9　肺动脉环缩+三腔起搏联合对抗小儿顽固性心力衰竭

注：a.术前心电图（完全性左束支传导阻滞）；b.术前超声显示左室扩张；c.术后超声；d.手术中。

Figure 2-9　Pulmonary artery banding combined with three-chamber pacemaker against heart failure in children

a. preoperative electrocardiogram (compelete left bundle branch black); b.preoperative altrasound showed left ventricular dilatation; c.postoperative ultrasound; d.intraoperative photo.

肺静脉支架联合西罗莫司治疗肺静脉狭窄
Pulmonary vein stent combined with sirolimus in the treatment of pulmonary vein stenosis

　　3岁男性患儿，诊断为肺静脉狭窄，经历过两次经皮肺静脉球囊扩张术，左上、左下、右上三支狭窄的肺静脉引起肺动脉压继发升高，多次大量咯血，使用成人IBS可吸收药物洗脱冠脉支架，并给予西罗莫司抑制肺静脉内膜增生（图2-10）。

A 3-year-old male child was diagnosed with pulmonary vein stenosis and underwent two percutaneous balloon dilatation of the pulmonary vein. The stenosis of the left- superior, left-inferior and right-superior pulmonary veins increased pulmonary artery pressure and caused massive hemoptysis. Coronary stents were covered with adult IBS absorbable eluted drugs, and sirolimus was given to inhibit pulmonary vein intimal hyperplasia (Figure 2-10).

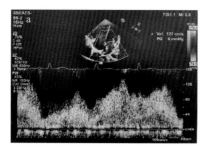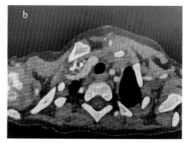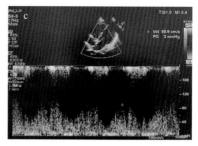

图2-10　肺静脉支架联合西罗莫司治疗肺静脉狭窄

注：a. 治疗前前肺静脉血流流速高；b. 增强CT；c. 治疗后肺静脉血流流速显著降低。

Figure 2-10　Pulmonary vein stent combined with sirolimus in the treatment of pulmonary vein stenosis

a. Before treatment, the flow speed of pulmonary vein was high; b. CTA; c. The flow velocity of pulmonary vein decreased significantly after treatment.

OUTCOMES 2022

心血管康复医疗

CARDIOVASCULAR REHABILITATION

一、外科围手术期的全程康复
Rehabilitation in perioperative period of surgery

心脏康复贯穿于心脏外科围手术期的全周期。从患者入院，即开始预康复，进行肢体活动和呼吸训练，提高术前身体功能，减少ICU获得性虚弱，降低气管插管时间。患者手术后，从ICU住院期就开始早期评估及康复训练，降低术后并发症，减少住院时间。转回病房后，患者将继续延续康复训练，逐步提高活动水平，直至出院。出院前给予患者的评估结果，将指导患者的过渡期康复。术后3个月，患者可至心脏康复门诊开展以运动、营养、睡眠、呼吸、心理为核心的二期康复，优化患者的体能和身体状态，完成疾病的二级预防，提高生活质量，并终身保持健康生活方式（图3-1）。

Cardiac rehabilitation runs through the perioperative cycle of cardiac surgery. From the time the patients were admitted, they undertook pre-rehabilitation, physical training and breathing training to improve the physical function before operation, reduce the acquired weakness of ICU and shorten tracheal intubation time. After operation, the patients undertook early evaluation and rehabilitation training in ICU to reduce postoperative complications and hospitalization time. After being transferred back to the ward, the patients will continue their rehabilitation training and gradually improve their activity level until they are discharged. The evaluation results given to the patients before discharge will guide the patients' transitional recovery. Three months after operation, patients can go to the cardiac rehabilitation clinic to carry out second-stage rehabilitation with exercise, nutrition, sleep, breathing, and psychology, optimize their physical fitness and physical condition, complete the secondary prevention of the disease, improve their quality of life. and maintain a healthy lifestyle (Figure 3-1).

2022年，心脏康复中心将心外科围手术期康复拓展到成人外科病房、血管外科病房、结构病房、小儿外科病房、外科术后ICU等12个病区，指导了包括心脏搭桥、瓣膜置换、人工血管置换、先心病手术、心脏移植、经皮瓣膜手术、左心室辅助术等外科手术患者的康复，提供共计51 456人次的外科住院康复，康复量较2019年提高了90%。门诊康复共计6106人次，较2019年提高147%（图3-2）。心脏康复中心病房为患者提供肺康复、徒手康复、踏车训练、肌力评估和肺功能评估项目，2022年总计完成康复和评估项目52 896人次（图3-3）。

In 2022, the Cardiac Rehabilitation Center expanded the perioperative rehabilitation of cardiac surgery to 12 wards to guide the rehabilitation of patients undergoing surgery, including coronary artery bypass grafting, valve replacement, congenital heart disease surgery, heart transplantation, percutaneous valve surgery, and LVAD surgery. 51,456 patients undertook rehabilitation, with an increase of 90% over 2019. The total number of outpatient rehabilitation

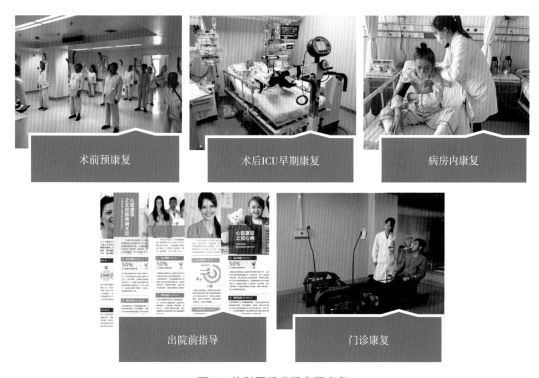

术前预康复

术后ICU早期康复

病房内康复

出院前指导

门诊康复

图3-1 外科围手术期全程康复

Figure 3-1 Perioperative rehabilitation of surgery

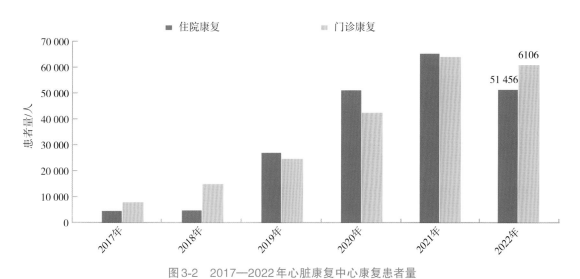

图3-2　2017—2022年心脏康复中心康复患者量

Figure 3-2 The volume of patients in cardiac rehabilitation centers in 2017—2022

was 6106, with an increase of 147% over 2019 (Figure 3-2). The cardiac rehabilitation center provides patients with lung rehabilitation, unarmed rehabilitation, treadmill training, muscle strength assessment and lung function assessment. 52,896 rehabilitation and assessment were completed in 2022 (Figure 3-3).

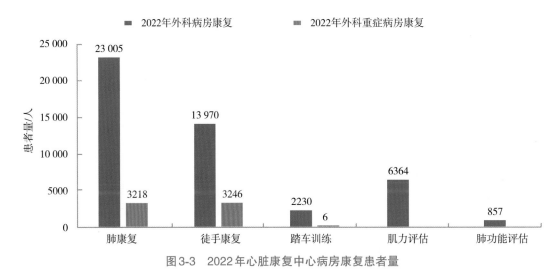

图3-3　2022年心脏康复中心病房康复患者量

Figure 3-3 The volume of patients in the cardiac rehabilitation center ward in 2022

二、特色门诊
Featured clinic

2022年，心脏康复中心开展了与临床工作紧密联系的特色门诊，从多个维度满足临床患者需求（图3-4）。

营养门诊：可通过膳食调查，体成分分析，代谢车测量代谢水平等方式，评估患者的营养状况，制定个性化饮食方案，防止总热量摄入过多或各种营养素之间的不平衡等因素造成心血管疾病风险。

中西医结合门诊：通过传统中医手段（如太极、八段锦、针灸、拔罐等），结合经典心脏康复治疗方式（如运动、营养等），为患者提供多元化的中西医结合的心脏康复干预方案。

双心门诊：由心理团队和心内科团队共同组成的双心门诊，服务心血管疾病合并精神心理障碍的患者。在筛查心脏疾病的同时，可通过精神药物及心理咨询、生物反馈等治疗方式，对患者的精神心理问题进行同步诊疗。

In 2022, the Cardiac Rehabilitation Center launched featured clinic to help clinical patients（Figure 3-4）.

Nutrition clinic: through dietary survey, body composition analysis and metabolic vehicle measurement of metabolic level, nutrition clinic evaluates the nutritional status of patients and offers a personalized diet plan to prevent excessive calorie intake or imbalance between various nutrient, which reduce cardiovascular risk.

Traditional Chinese and western medicine integrated clinic: traditional Chinese medicine (such as Taiji, Baduanjin and other traditional sports, acupuncture, cupping, etc.) combined with classical cardiac rehabilitation treatment (such as exercise, nutrition, etc.), provides patients with a variety of cardiac rehabilitation programs.

Combined clinic: a combined clinic composed of psychological team and cardiology team to serve patients with both cardiovascular disease and mental disorders. Patients mental and psychological problems can be diagnosed and treated synchronously through psychotropic drugs, psychological counseling or other non-drug treatment.

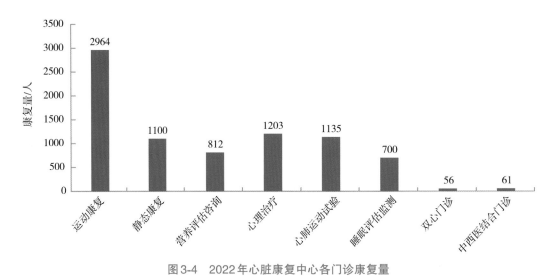

图3-4　2022年心脏康复中心各门诊康复量

Figure 3-4 The volume of out-patients in the cardiac rehabilitation clinic in 2022

▶ **自主研发优势，打造线上线下一体化的就医体验**
Integrated online and offline medical treatment

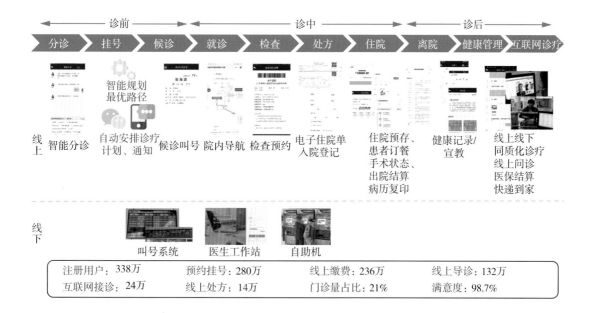

| 注册用户：338万 | 预约挂号：280万 | 线上缴费：236万 | 线上导诊：132万 |
| 互联网接诊：24万 | 线上处方：14万 | 门诊量占比：21% | 满意度：98.7% |

▶ **就诊后：患者健康改善计划平台**
Post-clinic: Health improvement plan

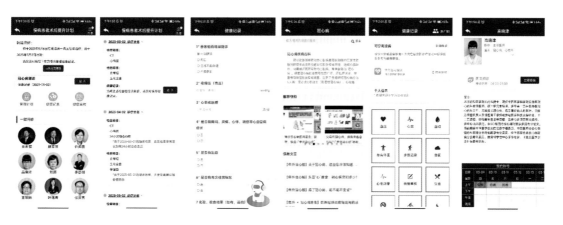

患者健康改善计划平台上线，提升院后健康管理服务能力

➢ 一部手机随时随地线上诊疗，打破诊疗空间和时间。

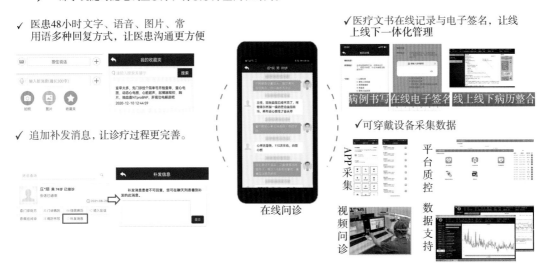

✓ 医患48小时文字、语音、图片、常用语多种回复方式，让医患沟通更方便

✓ 追加补发消息，让诊疗过程更完善。

在线问诊

✓ 医疗文书在线记录与电子签名，让线上线下一体化管理

病例书写 在线电子签名 线上线下病历整合

✓ 可穿戴设备采集数据

APP采集　平台质控

视频问诊　数据支持

▶ **线上线下数据全打通，集成到手机为医师诊疗提供更全面的参考与支持**
Doctors can acquire patients medical data online.

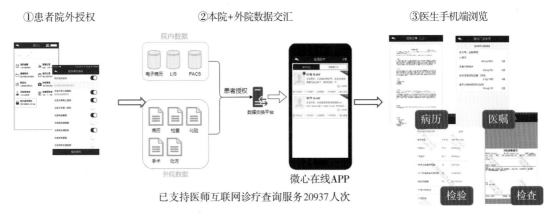

①患者院外授权　　②本院+外院数据交汇　　③医生手机端浏览

院内数据

电子病历　LIS　PACS

患者授权

数据交换平台

微心在线APP

已支持医师互联网诊疗查询服务20937人次

病历　检查　化验

手术　处方

外院数据

病历　医嘱

检验　检查

医师线上诊疗可查看患者本院及外院的门诊/急诊/住院病历、医嘱、检查、检验的全量数据

OUTCOMES 2022

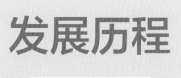

发展历程

HISTORY

1956年，阜外医院的前身——中国人民解放军胸科医院于黑山扈成立。

In 1956, the predecessor of Fuwai Hospital, the Chest Hospital of the Chinese People s Liberation Army (PLA), was founded in the Heishanhu area of Beijing.

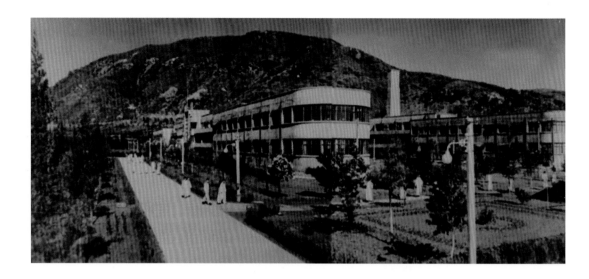

1958年，中国人民解放军胸科医院移交地方，迁至阜成门外，归属中国医学科学院，更名为中国医学科学院阜成门外医院，简称"阜外医院"。

In 1958, responsibility for the Chest Hospital of Chinese PLA was transferred to the local government. The hospital was subsequently relocated to Fuchengmenwai Street, became affiliated with the Chinese Academy of Medical Sciences, and was renamed Fuchengmenwai Hospital Affiliated to the Chinese Academy of Medical Sciences, or Fuwai Hospital for short.

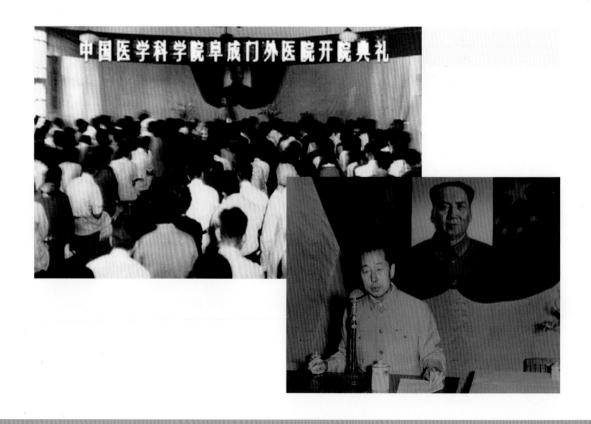

1962年，阜外医院兼称心脏血管系统疾病研究所，形成院所一体化的心血管病专科医院。
In 1962, Fuwai Hospital was designated as an Institute for Cardiovascular Diseases, identifying it as a hospital specializing in cardiovascular diseases that integrates both patient care and medical research.

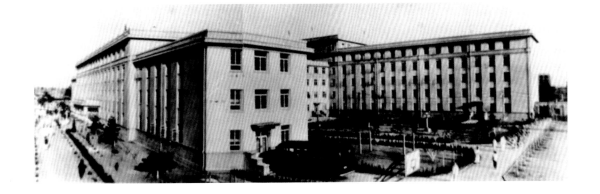

1994年，中国医学科学院阜外医院更名为中国医学科学院阜外心血管病医院。
In 1994, Fuwai Hospital Affiliated to the Chinese Academy of Medical Sciences was renamed Fuwai Cardiovascular Hospital, Chinese Academy of Medical Sciences.

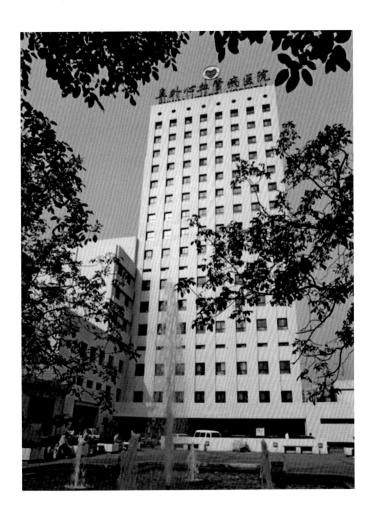

2004年，卫生部心血管病防治研究中心成立，标志着我院成为集医疗、科研、教学、预防为一体的国家级心血管病专科医院。

In 2004, the Cardiovascular Disease Prevention, Treatment and Research Center affiliated to the Ministry of Health was established, marking the official recognition of our hospital as a national institution specializing in cardiovascular disease and integrating medical care, scientific research, medical education, and disease prevention.

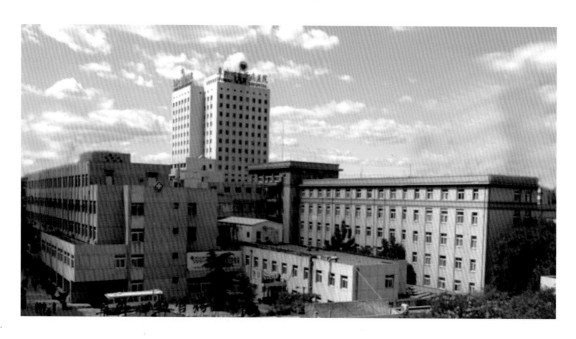

2011年，心血管疾病国家重点实验室落户阜外医院。

In 2011, the State Key Laboratory of Cardiovascular Diseases joined Fuwai Hospital.

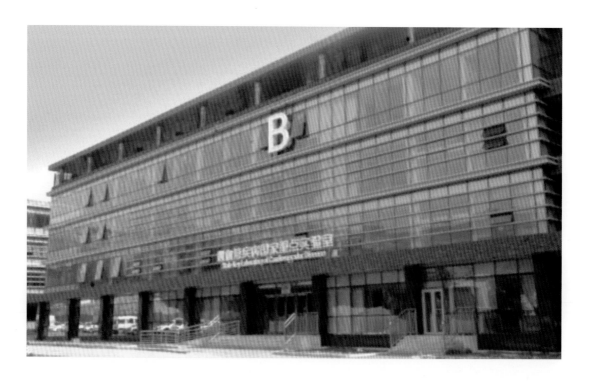

科学技术部文件

科技发基〔2011〕317号

关于批准建设心血管疾病等
49 个国家重点实验室的通知

北京市、天津市、辽宁省、吉林省、黑龙江省、上海市、江苏省、浙江省、福建省、河南省、湖北省、湖南省、广东省、广西壮族自治区、重庆市、四川省、甘肃省、新疆维吾尔自治区科技厅（委），教育部、工业和信息化部、国土资源部、环境保护部、水利部、卫生部、中国科学院、中国地震局、中国气象局、中国人民解放军总后勤部卫生部。

根据《国家重点实验室建设与运行管理办法》（国科发基〔2008〕539号）有关要求，结合我国经济社会与科学技术发展需要，对依托有关单位建设的心血管疾病等49 个国家重点实验室建设计划任务书进行了审核批准。

2013年，阜外医院西山科研基地全面启用。
In 2013, the Xishan scientific research base was fully launched.

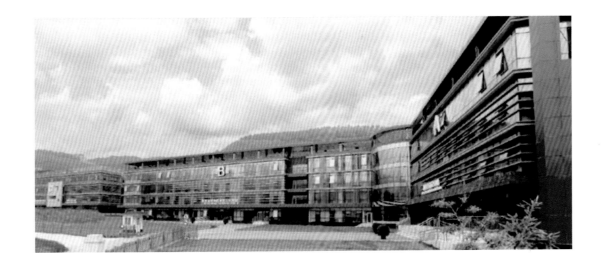

中共国家卫生和计划生育委员会党组文件

国卫党任发〔2013〕17号

中共国家卫生和计划生育委员会党组
关于胡盛寿、李惠君同志任职的通知

国家心血管病中心：

经委党组研究决定，任命：

胡盛寿同志为国家心血管病中心主持工作的副主任；

李惠君同志为国家心血管病中心副主任。

以上同志按规定实行任职试用期制。

中　　　　　　　　　　党
国家卫生和计划生育委员会党组
201 年9月 日

2013年，国家心血管疾病临床医学研究中心落户阜外医院。
In 2013, the National Clinical Research Center for Cardiovascular Diseases joined Fuwai Hospital.

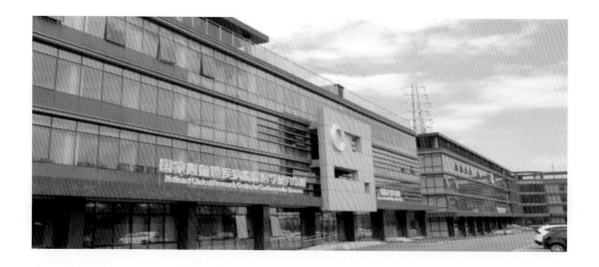

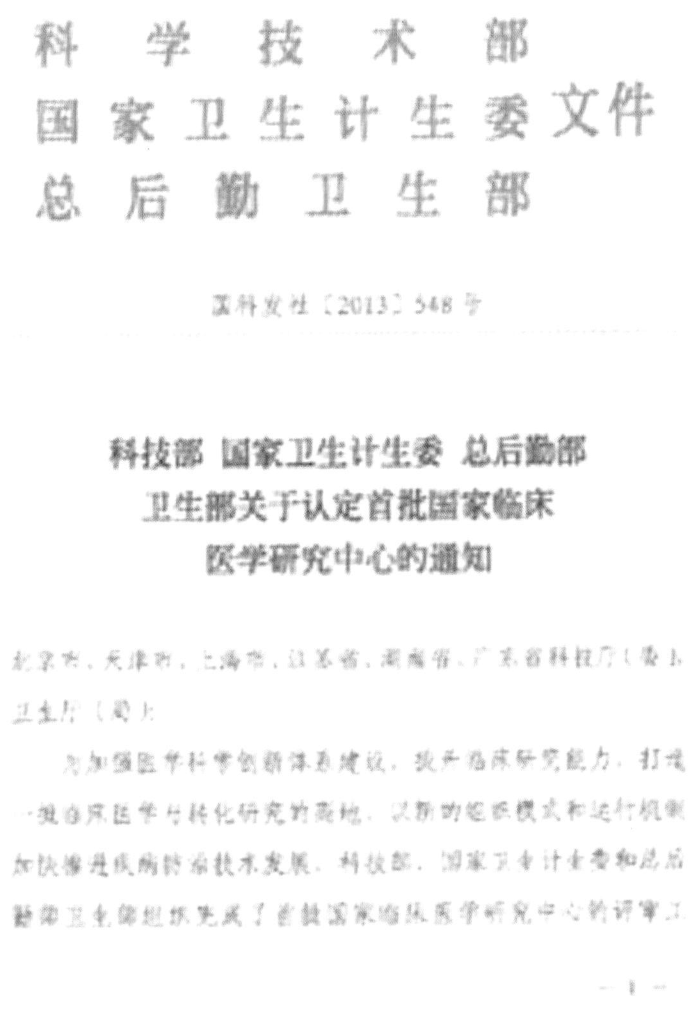

科 学 技 术 部
国 家 卫 生 计 生 委 文件
总 后 勤 卫 生 部

国科发社〔2013〕548号

科技部 国家卫生计生委 总后勤部
卫生部关于认定首批国家临床
医学研究中心的通知

北京市、天津市、上海市、江苏省、湖南省、广东省科技厅（委）、
卫生厅（局）：

为加强医学科学创新体系建设，提升临床研究能力，打造
一批临床医学与转化研究的高地，以新的组织模式和运行机制
加快推进疾病防治技术发展，科技部、国家卫生计生委和总后
勤部卫生部组织完成了首批国家临床医学研究中心的评审工

— 1 —

　　2014年，中国医学科学院阜外心血管病医院更名为中国医学科学院阜外医院。国家心血管病中心和中国医学科学院阜外医院正式进入"两个独立法人，一套行政机构"两位一体的运行模式。

In 2014, Fuwai Cardiovascular Hospital, Chinese Academy of Medical Sciences was renamed Fuwai Hospital, Chinese Academy of Medical Sciences, National Center for Cardiovascular Disease. The hospital began operating under the dual integrated operation model, which is based on the "two independent legal persons, one administration system."

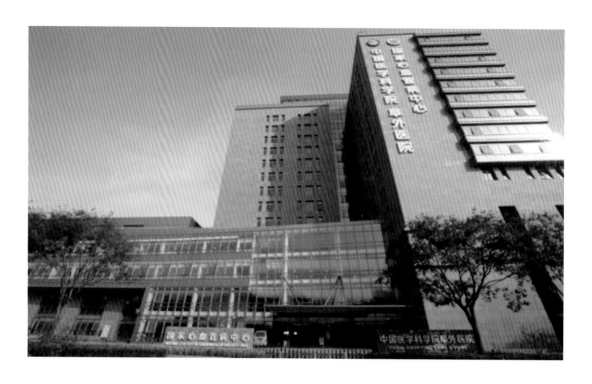

　　2015年，阜外医院正式启用了集门诊、急诊、住院、手术等为一体的综合大楼，目前已成为世界上最大的心血管疾病诊治中心和集医疗、科研、预防和人才培养于一体的国家级医学研究与教育中心。

In 2015, the new medical building opened, integrating the clinic, emergency, and surgical systems to efficiently serve an even greater number of patients. The center has become the world s largest cardiovascular center as well as a national cardiovascular center for treatment, prevention, and medical research and education.

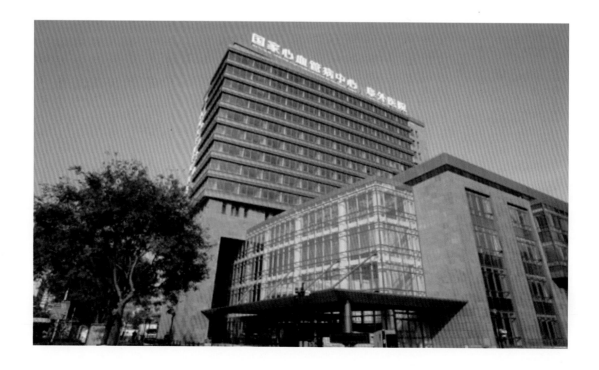